METAMORPHOSES

Metamorphoses

MEMOIRS OF A LIFE IN MEDICINE

William G. Anlyan, M.D.

To Bettye
With profound appreciation
for our longtime friendship
and mutual interests
Fondly
Bill
Aug 17/04

DUKE UNIVERSITY PRESS *Durham and London 2004*

© 2004 Duke University Press
All rights reserved
Printed in the United States of America on acid-free paper ∞
Typeset in Galliard by Tseng Information Systems, Inc.
Library of Congress Cataloging-in-Publication Data appear
on the last printed page of this book.

This book is dedicated to all future
students embarking on careers in
health. An exciting field in my own time,
it promises to be no less exciting
in the lives of generations to come.

Metamorphoses in aeternum

Contents

Illustrations

Figures

Prologue

IN THIS MEMOIR, I look back at a life in medicine, one that has been characterized by enormous changes in my personal life and in the life of the institutions, the cities, and the world in my lifetime. Many of these changes came from outside, but some I hope I can claim as personal accomplishments.

The Medical School and Hospital at Duke University, under my watch, changed from being a small and relatively unknown regional school to becoming one of the top institutions in the country. We became organized as a corporation, with all our different elements and personnel working together as one organization. It was not an autocracy, because I firmly believed that it was important to make decisions with the support of the corporate leadership. On the other hand, it was also important to know when some decisions needed to be made at the top, as in the building of the new hospital. There is an art to knowing what to bring to a vote, when to bring it to a vote, and how to manage it.

The other thing I might have accomplished is to help foster a sense of corporate responsibility at the top level by recruiting a number of outstanding department chairmen as leaders and establishing a Medical School advisory committee. I succeeded in getting the hospital and clinic operations under an M.D., so that that person, along with the clinical chairmen, could work on the day-to-day problems of the hospital. After defining the relationship of the Private Diagnostic Clinics to the hospital, the Medical School and university, I left the PDCs largely alone for the clinical chairmen to manage.

I built a superlative staff of people to do the nonmedical business of the

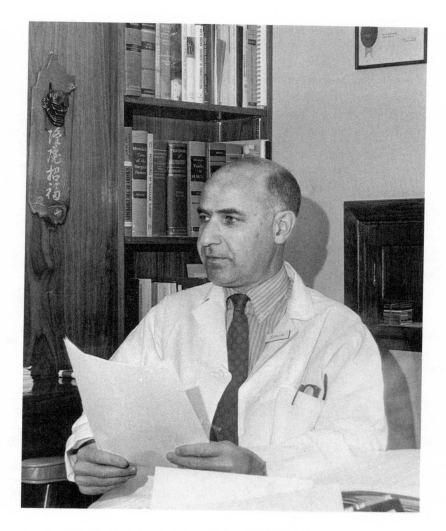

1   Dr. William G. Anlyan, third dean of the Duke University
School of Medicine. DUMC Photography.

medical center. I knew that I was not trained in business management and
that I was therefore going to depend on people who were, who could keep
an eye on the business and financial management of the institution.

I have been fortunate also to be involved in medical organizations outside of Duke in professional societies and groups such as the AAMC and

AAHC and the National Library of Medicine, work that has taken me all over the country and the world. More recently, I have served in various capacities in organizations such as Research!America and The Duke Endowment, drawing on my long career at the helm of the Duke Medical Center. In this book, I hope to show the route my path has taken, beginning when I was a schoolboy in Alexandria, Egypt, and reaching to the present, at the start of a new century in North Carolina.

Acknowledgments

THESE MEMOIRS RECALL with gratitude my parents, Armand and Emmy Anlyan, whose commitment to high-quality education and hard work were the roadway for me and my brothers, John and Fred. I have also been blessed with three wonderful children: Bill Jr., Pete, and Louise, and their families. I credit their mother, Connie, for their admirable traits. Not least, I thank my wife, Alex, who for ten years has been my partner in multiple enjoyable endeavors, adapting with grace to my septuagenarian years.

I would like to acknowledge Joyce Ruark, my devoted secretary and assistant for nearly thirty years, for taking such personal care of many aspects of my activities and for her tremendous assistance in collecting and organizing years of historical data for my memoirs. I also want to recognize the editorial assistance of Edith Roberts, Maura High, and Ginna Davidson.

It is a pleasure also to acknowledge my special friendship with Mary Biddle Duke Trent Semans, over the fifty-five years I have been at Duke. Mary, a Duke trustee, and chairman for many years of The Duke Endowment, has been a key person in the development of many programs at Duke and in North Carolina. She and her husband, Jim, have been two of the most important supporters of philanthropy in the state. I have also especially enjoyed working with President Doug Knight (who appointed me dean of the Medical School in 1963) and President Terry Sanford, who, with Alex McMahon, were such stronger supporters of the evolutions of the Medical Center.

Many friends and colleagues have played an important role in my life;

so many, in fact, that it is not possible to name them all here, though some are referred to in this text. I do, however, express my particular gratitude to the following: my personal friends Ruth and Nick Georgiade, Georgia and Roy Parker, Ort and Bud Busse and their families, who grew up with my children; my classmates at Victoria College, many of whom are still alive and scattered throughout the world in the United States, Canada, the United Kingdom, and the Middle East; the Yale class of 1945W, many of whom, because of World War II, didn't meet until our reunion years; my Yale Medical School class of 1949, a great group of individuals that I was fortunate enough to know each member of—many of them are alive today following retirement; and Duke medical alumni who have been gracious and supportive, including those who preceded my arrival in 1949 and especially those who were students or fellow residents from 1949 to 1955 and who served with me "in the trenches." During my administrative phase I got to know especially well the student leaders and those who were courageous enough to pick me as their tennis partner.

Finally, it is important to recognize the peace of mind I have had in collaborating with my successor, Ralph Snyderman, during his successful and constructive fifteen-year tenure at the helm of the Duke Medical Center. Mine was the golden age of medicine; Ralph steered the ship during some very challenging years.

METAMORPHOSES

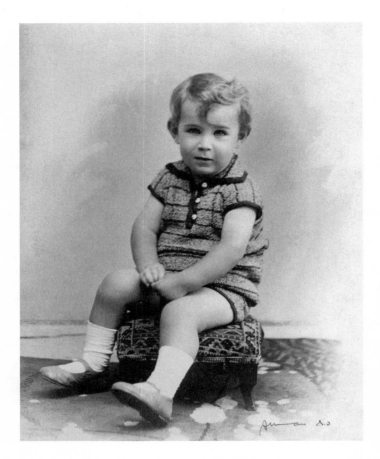

2   Dr. W. G. Anlyan as a young child, before *Metamorphoses*.
From personal archive of author.

I

THE ROAD TO NORTH CAROLINA

I WAS BORN IN Alexandria, in the British protectorate of Egypt, on October 14, 1925, the second of three sons of Armenian parents. My mother and father had both grown up in Alexandria, in families that had left Turkey in the late nineteenth century. My mother's grandparents came from the town of Ayinkaf; my father's grandfather, from Diyarbakir. He had left in 1873, in the waning years of the Ottoman Empire, bringing with him his two sons and their families. The younger son went to Boston; the elder stayed in Alexandria with his father, where he set up business in textiles and proved a shrewd businessman.

Growing up in such an environment, at such a point in history, would leave its mark on anyone, and I was no exception. Alexandria was a cosmopolitan city with a rich history and a vibrant cultural life. We lived in the suburb of Ibrahimieh in a comfortable villa with grounds ample enough to accommodate flower gardens, our own little vineyard and vegetable garden, servants quarters, garages, and storage sheds. My paternal grandparents lived on the second floor in their own apartment and went about their own business, joining us for meals only on special holidays. In 1939, when the Second World War broke out, I was a schoolboy, attending Victoria College, a British school that had been founded in 1901, the year of Queen Victoria's death.[1] My schoolmates included the sons of British families

---

1. "Although the school may have been started primarily for the British, there was an immediate understanding implicit in the fact that it was free from consular, community, and church control; and, perhaps most important, since it was established as a business venture, it would be open to

living in the Middle East and the scions of prominent families from Egypt to Singapore: princes from Ethiopia, Iraq, and Jordan, and the son of the prime minister of Egypt, who once invited me to watch the fireworks celebrating the marriage of King Farouk to the shah of Iran's daughter from the balcony of the San Stefano Hotel.

My father, Armand Anlyan, was an intellectual at heart. Born in 1892 in Alexandria and educated in a Swiss school in Alexandria, he had wanted to be a physician but ended up, like his own father, in commerce. We children were not privy to the family's financial matters, but I suspect my father was not an adept businessman. On one occasion my frugal grandfather told me that his son had learned only to spend money. My father was not a communicative man, and we did not see very much of him. I once asked him what it was that he did, and he told me it was none of my business. He was, however, interested in making sure his sons got a good education and worked diligently at school. If we earned less than an A in any course, we had to answer to him. He also believed we should develop physical stamina, making us get up at six every morning. We jumped rope and took turns at boxing with him, and he usually beat us hands down. I learned many years later that he had worked for British Intelligence during the war. Because he was fluent in German and could tell which region of Germany someone came from just from the person's accent and choice of words, he was assigned to debrief captured German Army and Luftwaffe personnel and to pick up German spies who tried to pass themselves off as Afrikaners. Once, when the city was threatened with attack, he asked me to help him burn his files, though I did not know what they contained and did not dare ask.

My mother, Emmy Nazaretian, was born in 1900, in Alexandria, like my father, and, like my father, was educated in French schools in Alexandria. Though we used English and French at home, my mother would speak Turkish to our cook, colloquial Arabic to the other servants, and Armenian with her older relatives, often mixed with English, Turkish, or French, adding to the multiplicity of languages around us. I learned classical Arabic at school partly at her insistence, in case I ended up remaining in Egypt. I saw more of my mother than I did of my father, mainly because she moni-

all. And so it was. It attracted the children of royalty, dignitaries, diplomats, magnates, ministers, political refugees, landowners, and very ordinary people. It educated children of all nationalities, not only from all over Egypt, but also from the entire Middle East and beyond. Victoria College gained a reputation that made it the foremost school in the Middle East." Sahar Hamouda and Colin Clement, *Victoria College: A History Revealed* (Cairo: American University in Cairo Press, 2002).

tored our musical education: the violin for my older brother, John, and the piano for Fred and me. Music had figured largely in her own life, at least as a social accomplishment: she and her sisters, Lucy and Rose, had been expected to supply the after-dinner entertainment in their family's home, singing and playing the piano for guests. For a while, my family nurtured the hope that I might become a concert pianist, and for two or three hours a day I would practice under my mother's supervision, even though I could hardly reach the pedals and keyboard. While my friends were playing outdoors, I had to work on my exercises, with tears rolling down my cheeks (according to my older brother, John, who was able to give up the violin when his teacher said that the family was wasting its resources in teaching him music). Other than these occasional interventions in our education, my mother's main interests were those of a society woman. In August 1938, when I was a teenager, she preceded John to the United States, where he was bound for Yale University. She took my younger brother, Fred, with her, and they stayed in New Haven with her sister, Rose, and her family for almost two years.

It was in many ways an extraordinary and privileged childhood, and not an unhappy one, despite the emotional distance of my parents and grandparents, despite the enforced boxing and music lessons and the pressure on us to succeed in school, despite being the second son, living always in the shadow of my older brother, John. I learned to swim and in the summer months swam for hours in the Mediterranean. My mother's brother, George, and his wife, Agnes, from Holland, included me in many gatherings. I learned to enjoy music and looked forward to my lessons with Maestro Amideus Bottari, our Neapolitan piano teacher. At the age of fourteen, when I was preparing to play Tchaikovsky's Piano Concerto no. 1 in B-flat minor, I realized that I just did not have enough talent to tackle it, and I abandoned the idea of becoming a professional pianist. But I never lost my interest in music and widened it to include modern music and musical shows, performing in and directing musical events at school and beyond.

School also interested me, and I still remember clearly many of my teachers and the lessons they taught me, passages memorized from Shakespeare, Chaucer, the history of Europe and America from the British perspective, the caning I got from the headmaster, Mr. Reed, for some infraction I no longer recall, my year as head boy (following in the footsteps of John), our stints as troop leaders in the Boy Scouts and later as assistant scoutmasters (it was in the Scouts that I learned to tie a square knot, later so useful to me in surgery). I graduated in 1943 with my Oxford and Cambridge Higher

Certificate in physics, chemistry, and biology, and was set to follow John to Yale, as soon as the passage could be arranged to America.

The war marked a turning point in our lives, but living as we did in Alexandria, we were sheltered from its worst effects. Victoria College was converted into a military hospital, wooden buildings were erected on the soccer fields to accommodate the wounded soldiers, and the school moved into the San Stefano Hotel, from where I had watched the fireworks only a few years before. We moved out of our large villa into an apartment in Cleopatra, another suburb of the city, just one mile from the British Army headquarters at Sidi Gaber. My mother and two brothers were still in the United States when the first enemy air raids rattled the city, in May 1940. They were carried out by the Italian Air Force, which never penetrated the airspace over Alexandria but dropped their bombs over the Mediterranean and then flew back to their base in Libya. In June 1941, however, the Luftwaffe took over from the Italians, and for the first time, the bombs came close. We took these raids seriously and would go down to the air raid shelter when the alarm sounded. From then on, we had air raids most evenings for two years. The Germans were systematic—in general the raids began one hour after the moon rose, so you could plan your social life ahead. The nearest bomb to where we lived fell half a mile away, jolting our building but hurting no one. You learned to move in the dark without streetlights and to drive without headlights. All the houses had heavy curtains. In August of 1942 my father was monitoring Radio Berlin, and I remember distinctly hearing the announcement "Alexandrie ist gefallen." We expected at any moment that Hitler's Afrika Korps, commanded by the charismatic General Rommel, would come rolling in. They never came: General Montgomery had routed the German forces at the battle of El Alamein, and life in the city returned to its peacetime rhythms.

Sometime in the summer of 1943 my father received a call from the U.S. War Shipping Administration in Cairo to say that I would be given a passage to the United States on a U.S. merchant vessel in late August. I was to "disappear," without letting anyone know where I was going or why, and report to Port Said, at the north end of the Suez Canal, to wait further instructions. Because I was under eighteen years old, my parents were, to my great relief, allowed to accompany me. So, without farewells to friends and other relatives, we left, by train from Alexandria, changing once in the town of Tanta.

The Port Said harbor was filled with large numbers of ships, including British warships. My parents and I assumed I would be assigned to a convoy going down the canal to the Indian Ocean and around the Cape of Good Hope, on a slow voyage to an unknown destination in the United States. The plan was for me to find my way to New Haven, where I would join my brother John at Yale. Port Said had no historic sites or museums and only one large trading store, so the days of waiting seemed interminable and dull. I found a small spinet piano in the hotel and kept busy playing from the sheet music and albums I had brought with me to take to the United States. After five days, my father got word that I was to be at a certain dock at a specified time, ready to embark on the U.S. liberty ship SS *Louis Hennepin*. My father gave me a money belt containing five thousand dollars, which I was to keep on me or within direct vision at all times. So we said our goodbyes at the dockside, and I boarded the ship. This voyage was going to be very different from the one my brother took in 1939, in a comfortable cabin aboard the passenger ship SS *President Wilson* of the President Lines.

The *Hennepin* had been built by the Kaiser Company, and, although rumored to be structurally weak, it was commissioned to deliver military supplies from San Francisco to support the Pacific war. Having delivered its cargo in Australia, it was now making its way home to the United States. Its captain, Captain Simon, had been master of a dynamite barge in the Gulf of Mexico before being given command of the *Hennepin*. I was assigned to a cabin with three junior officers and, as the only civilian aboard, was to have the privilege of sitting at the captain's table in the officer's dining room. The ship weighed anchor after I fell asleep. When I awoke the next morning, much to my surprise, I saw the Mediterranean beaches of Egypt instead of the Red Sea. That afternoon, we docked in Alexandria; I was overcome by homesickness and had to fight back the temptation to find the captain and ask to disembark and be returned to my family and friends.

The next morning we set sail once again, part of a sixty-ship convoy that would be the first to cross the Mediterranean in wartime by hugging the coastline of North Africa. A British destroyer escort of First World War vintage crisscrossed the waters at the head of the convoy, which was moving at about seven and a half knots. On either side were several tugboats that would occasionally drop depth charges to "neutralize" enemy submarines lurking nearby. With the help of the *Hennepin*'s first officer, Commander Anderson, I moved to a single cabin, the deck engineer's cabin behind the engine room. The engineer was apparently in the brig, for reasons that were never clear to me. The cabin was very hot, and the portholes were sealed because of blackout restrictions. But I remembered from my physics class that white sheets hung in the doorway would deflect some of the heat, and that helped.

Four days out of Alexandria, a general alert was sounded. We donned life jackets and reported to our lifeboats; the fifty U.S. naval personnel on board to protect the ship went to battle stations. About twenty-five minutes after the alert, we learned that the bulk of the Italian Navy was heading straight toward us. The good news was that they were on their way to surrender in the Port of Tunis, thus ending their participation in the war. Battleships, cruisers, destroyers, and a couple of aircraft carriers, steamed by our port side. The men crowded on their decks were waving and cheering as they sailed past, music was playing loudly; the Italians were clearly overjoyed to be going out of the war.

After four more days, we dropped anchor in Gibraltar Bay, among hundreds of other warships and transports, in a vast enclosure bounded by anti-submarine netting. We remained there for six days awaiting the formation of our transatlantic convoy, under the watchful eyes of the German consulate, which was strategically located on a hillside in Algeciras, Spain, overlooking the entire bay. Each night, British patrol boats moved among the ships and dropped small depth charges to prevent anti-Allied divers from attaching suction bombs to the hulls of the anchored ships. With the exception of Captain Simon, no one had shore leave. On the third day, the captain decided to run an abandon ship drill. After the incident with the Italian Navy, I had been wondering how the lifeboat and safety systems worked, and now I was to learn. He sounded the signal, and I reported to my assigned lifeboat, number 3. We got in, but the pulleys to lower the boat did not work. Ninety minutes later, we finally came down to the level of the water, and the ropes to the pulleys were disconnected. No one had considered that this would set us adrift. For the next thirty minutes, the third mate, Mr. Pollard, tried in vain to start the inboard motor engine. When Pollard finally commanded, "Man the oars," two of the sailors muttered, "What?" They had never been in a rowboat before. Finally, a British patrol boat arrived to tow us back to the *Hennepin*, where the captain was waiting to excoriate the third mate mercilessly and publicly. At that point, I decided that in the event of another abandon ship order, I would take a running dive off the side and swim as fast as I could.

In the late afternoon of the sixth day, we weighed anchor, along with dozens of other ships, all heading east. No one except the captain knew what our course would be. Were we going back to the eastern Mediterranean? If so, where? It was only the next morning that I discovered we had in the night slipped past the U-boats nested outside the Straits of Gibraltar and were in the middle of a 120-ship convoy, headed west, across the Atlantic Ocean. The convoy was commanded by a commodore, who was aboard a large U.S. destroyer that tacked back and forth at relatively high speed in front of the other ships. Several smaller destroyers and a converted aircraft carrier sailed alongside for protection, and we could watch reconnaissance aircraft coming in for landing and being snapped to a halt by "the hook." It felt good to be in the middle of the convoy. But our joy was short-lived. At noon on the first day, our captain ordered, "Stop the engines," causing the ships behind us to swerve right and left to avoid a collision. The captain was on the bridge with his rusty sextant (the first mate later told me he didn't know which end of the sextant was which), supposedly recording his ship's position, a function assumed in a convoy by the commodore. The commodore's vessel was blinking commands at a rapid pace. It took us until sundown to get back to our assigned positions in the convoy. The next day, precisely at noon, Captain Simon repeated his "Stop the engines" routine. More swerving of ships, more brisk signals from the commodore. By mid-afternoon, we were assigned a new position in the convoy: the back corner known as "torpedo junction." For the rest of our two-week journey, we stopped engines at noon, the sextant came out, and, by the time the captain was satisfied with his reading of our position, the rest of the convoy had disappeared over the horizon. We would then spend all night at full speed ahead to get back to torpedo junction. The commodore had clearly written us off.

The convoy managed to reach a point north of Bermuda unscathed. We were by then beginning to run out of food—the captain had somehow forgotten to reprovision in Gibraltar—and were eating potatoes twice a day. There was not much to do. The lounge on our ship was just the officers' dining room, and it was served by a very young cabin boy, who was so scared he never took off his life jacket. He did not know how to swim and was afraid of drowning. Everyone understood his situation, and nobody kidded him. I would tap out Chopin waltzes or Beethoven's Sonata no. 8 on the table when no one was watching.

At Bermuda, about half the ships turned north, while our half stayed on a course headed southwest. The U.S. Navy vessels accompanying us split evenly, with the aircraft carrier going north. Three days later, we entered Norfolk harbor through Hampton Roads, and I had my first view of my future homeland. I had grown so accustomed to the rolling and pitching of the ship that I walked very unsteadily onshore, as we made our way to the U.S. Customs house. The customs officers were clean-cut, polite young men in uniform, and the main thing they were concerned with was how much money was I carrying. I replied honestly, that I had five thousand dollars, to pay for my tuition and living expenses at Yale and was very surprised to be told by the head customs officer that I was allowed to bring in only fifty dollars. I would have to petition through the courts for the remainder of the money. There was no recourse. So I accepted a receipt for the confiscated money, took my two large suitcases, and followed directions to the railway station.

I was to take the overnight train to New York. The coaches were crowded with young men and women in uniform, but I found a free seat, and fell asleep. I was awoken at dawn by the trainman yelling, "Noo-werk, Noo-werk." I grabbed my bags and got off the train, only to discover that we were not in New York but in Newark, New Jersey. I barely made it back on board. Arriving at last at Pennsylvania Station, I took a yellow cab to Grand Central Station, a trip that seemed marvelous to me. The skyscrapers were real! It was just like the movies. I was agog. At Grand Central, I found the track for New Haven and bought a ticket. I also found the Western Union office and wired my parents: "Arrived safely in New York. Headed to New Haven."

We were indeed lucky to have made the trip unharmed, in over thirty-two days at a pace of seven and a half to eight knots, under the stewardship of a less-than-competent captain. What I did not realize at the time was how worried my parents had been for me, and how relieved they must have been to receive my telegram. They had learned that about twenty out of the sixty ships in the northbound contingent had been sunk by U-boats and did not know which part of the convoy I had been in once it split north of Bermuda. I was told later that my father was sick and depressed to think he might have sent me to my death and that my mother was wailing that her son had become food for fish in the ocean.

As for the $4,950 confiscated by the U.S. Customs at Norfolk, having engaged New York City lawyers specializing in such matters, after a year I received 60 percent of the money; the remaining 40 percent went to the lawyers.

2

BECOMING A DOCTOR

BACK IN 1943 New Haven did not look quite as run-down as it did in the 1990s. Yale impressed me as having a beautiful setting, particularly at dusk, when the lights of the various colleges were on (a change from the blackout of Alexandria). I had about three or four weeks to get acquainted with my new surroundings before classes formally started in November. I went to see Dean Edward Noyes of the admissions office, who decided I should have advanced standing as a first-semester sophomore because I had passed the Oxford and Cambridge Higher Certificate. I was assigned to the class of 1945W, the only class at Yale to have the letter *W* after the class year (*W* standing for "war"). Because it was wartime, college was in session year-round, though not everyone could attend full-time, and some of my classmates came and went.

Since I was studying toward a bachelor of science degree, I was enrolled in the Sheffield Scientific School (as it turned out, we were the last class to be designated as part of that school). At the end of the first semester, Dean Warren of the Sheffield School called me in and said, "I think we made a mistake." I thought he might be putting me back, but instead he made me a second-semester junior. Victoria College had prepped me well: I received my B.S. magna cum laude after just fifteen months of study.

I had decided fairly early on to go into medicine, so I tailored my course of study accordingly. I took first-semester comparative anatomy, second-semester histology, organic chemistry for a full year, and advanced physics. We were required to take French and German, so I took advanced courses in French and the first two years of German.

Our professors were both brilliant and memorable. Second-semester histology was with Alexander Petrunkevitch, the famed arachnologist. A White Russian émigré, he knew every spider species in the world. In his laboratory he kept an assortment of black widow spiders, and he gave each one a name and handled them individually. At tea every afternoon, he would fondle his spiders in the presence of his students and visitors. In Dr. Stevens's organic chemistry, we had to synthesize aspirin "on a desert island," using one lump of coal. Henry Margenau, a German refugee, taught us physics through calculus. He and I had some friendly arguments about pronunciation, about how to pronounce the word "ebullition," for instance. One day he dragged me down to the Sterling Memorial Library to settle this once and for all. He went straight to the *Webster's*, while I went to the Oxford English Dictionary. We were both right, but he got the upper hand when he said, "In America, do as *Webster* says."

My biology professors were Dan Merriman, G. Evelyn Hutchinson, and John Spangler Nicholas. In Merriman's anatomy course I wrote a thesis on the osseous system of a very rare fish he had in the oceanographic lab. Hutchinson took only four or five students a semester for a series of seminars. When he was awarded an honorary degree at Duke some years ago, he reminded me that I was the only student in his career who turned in a senior thesis written in verse. (I earnestly hope that has been destroyed.) The embryologist John Spangler Nicholas was head of the Department of Zoology. I cleaned his rat cages in exchange for free meals at Timothy Dwight College. Every Friday, after I had cleaned the cage litter, I would treat myself to dinner at Mory's, since the smell of the traditional Friday baked fish at Timothy Dwight was quite unbearable.

Other faculty who made an impression on me included Felix Zweig, the associate dean of engineering, and Henry Peyre, the chairman of the French Department. Since I was bilingual, I took some of Monsieur Peyre's advanced courses in French literature, reading Corneille's and Racine's plays as well as the writings of Descartes. M. Peyre showed us a 1944 film of the liberation of Paris from the Nazis. I could not have imagined at that time that forty years later I would be a guest of the Aga Khan, housed in the suite of the same Paris hotel where the Nazi general commanding Paris had surrendered to the Allies.

Of course, Yale was not only work. They needed people who could carry a tune, so I was invited to join the Yale Glee Club, then under the leadership of Marshall Bartholomew. We had a great deal of fun giving concerts and joint presentations with women's colleges such as Sarah Lawrence, Smith, and Mount Holyoke. I also became a member of Phi Gamma Delta, which at Yale was called Vernon Hall. The fraternities were divided into two groups. The B.A. students could pledge what were called "junior fraternities," and they became eligible in their senior year for secret societies such as Skull and Bones. The B.S. fraternities were "final fraternities," meaning we were not eligible for the societies.

During my early months in undergraduate school I experienced severe back pain, a symptom that had first appeared when I was fourteen. My father had taken me to a variety of specialists in Alexandria, who were not able to make a diagnosis. At Yale I was eventually referred to Malcolm Eveleth, chief of orthopedics at the Yale Hospital. Without much hesitation, he diagnosed Marie Strumpell arthritis (ankylosing spondylitis) of the spine, hips, and shoulders. To get a second opinion on whether I would be able to survive medical school, Dr. Eveleth sent me to Dr. Smith-Peterson, an orthopedic surgeon at Mass General in Boston, who tried to discourage my doing anything so arduous. As I rode the New Haven Railroad train back to Yale, my attitude was "I'll show that SOB." Dr. Smith-Peterson was famous for inventing a metal pin to insert in fractured hips. Subsequently, he was noted for being orthopedic surgeon to Arthur Godfrey, the radio and TV star, best remembered for his playing of the ukelele and performing with the singer Perry Como.

During my undergraduate days, the back pain became so bad that it would take me twenty-five minutes to get out of bed and straighten up before I dressed and had breakfast. I had then to walk up Prospect Hill for a quarter of an hour to get to my chemistry laboratory. Dr. Eveleth gave me a fairly heavy steel brace to wear (a Taylor brace, I believe). It was fortuitous that my Uncle Haig was a metallurgist, because he devised a duraluminum brace that was much lighter and brought a great change in my lifestyle. It had the metal on the front rather than the back, which came in particularly handy during my second year at Yale Medical School, when our pathology professor, Dr. Milton Winternitz stood by the door after one of the gross pathology classes and punched everybody in the solar plexus. When he came to me, he punched right into the metal. He shrieked with pain, "What are you trying to do? Break my wrist?" When I got to Duke I had two of those duraluminum braces. On one occasion Dr. Deryl Hart, the chief of surgery, had back pain from standing up for long periods in the operating room, so I loaned him a brace; many months later I had to remind him to give it back to me because I needed the spare. I was in the brace until the late sixties, when my spine had fused itself by itself and I no longer needed the extra support.

Arthritis hardly changed my life style or curbed my social life or educational experiences. I did everything everybody else did, except that I couldn't participate in some sports. I missed swimming (and still do), because I had enjoyed freestyle swimming in the Mediterranean, but with an ankylosed back it is hard to crank your neck above the water. At Yale I played squash—a game played with the wrist, which wasn't so hard on my fused shoulders and hips. Later on I discovered that I could use an underhand serve at tennis, and tennis remains my sport to this day.

I never missed a single day of classes as an undergraduate or as a medical student because of pain. For many years I took three aspirins every three or four hours; on some occasions when the pain was more severe I took one-half grain of codeine, but even a half-grain had the effect of making me nauseous, so I only took it on rare occasions. Dr. Eveleth felt I might benefit from radiation therapy to the spine and hips, so twice a week I would go to New York City for treatments under Dr. Philip Wilson at the Hospital for Special Surgery. Today we know that the only end result of such therapy is to increase one's chances of leukemia sixfold. Every time I get a routine blood count, I thank the Lord when the results are normal.

I was lucky to be assigned to Timothy Dwight College when I entered Yale. "TD," as it was called, was one of the two "civilian" colleges. The other colleges housed navy V-12 students or ASTP (Army Special Training Program) students in the army. Silliman College, across Temple Street from TD, housed all the Air Force cadets and the Glenn Miller orchestra, whose members presumably were all Yale students. Every afternoon around 4:00 P.M., Glenn Miller and his orchestra would lead an Air Force cadet parade to the New Haven Green, to lower the U.S. flag. Then, from about 5:00 to 7:00 P.M., the band would play jazz in the Silliman lounge while the cadets ate dinner in the adjacent dining room. It would always end with Glenn Miller's signature song. Though I became familiar with Benny Goodman and the Dorsey brothers and their bands on occasional visits to New York City, Glenn Miller's was the band I knew best and it became part of my musical fabric. I was shocked when the news came that Miller had died in a plane crash, when his plane plunged into the English Channel. He was only forty years old at his death. Hearing his music today by bands that retain his musical style brings back fond memories.

Timothy Dwight was a friendly place to call home. The housemaster,

Fred Godley, and his wife, Nan, would serve Sunday tea in the master's house and organize frequent special events. Since I was an overseas student, they took special care of me. Mr. Godley was the lone surviving architect of the team that had planned Rockefeller Center in New York. The Godleys were both very aristocratic in their bearing, tall, and easy in their interactions with students. They were kind enough to house our dates from visiting colleges on weekends. (Nan Godley, their daughter, preceded me by a year at Yale Medical School. She inherited the charm and intelligence of her parents.)

Others at Yale who were especially welcoming to me included the university chaplain, Sidney Lovett, and his family. The Lovetts lived in a university home on Wall Street within a stone's throw of TD. Every Thanksgiving and Christmas they included me among the handful of other guests. Faculty fellows of Timothy Dwight were also always available at lunch or dinner in the college dining room. (I estimate that half of my undergraduate education at Yale was acquired through extracurricular contacts with Yale faculty.)

I did not know President Charles Seymour personally, but I often passed him on his way to his office when I was headed to my science classes on Hillhouse Avenue. He always tipped his fedora hat as he went by. The closest I came to Mr. Seymour was on the occasion that I was asked to greet his visitors at a reception at the president's house. I was standing next to him, inquiring the names of the arriving guests so I could present them to the president. One guest introduced himself as Paul Hindemith. Before I could say, "President Seymour, may I present Mr. Hindemith," there was a brisk exchange: "Hi, Paul," "Hi, Charlie." (I learned from that episode never to use aides to introduce people in the receiving line but instead to rely on nametags large enough to be seen across the room. They would be color-coded to differentiate people from different groups—older-looking medical students, for example, from younger-looking faculty—and they had to be subtle: dark blue and black, rather than red and green. It never fails to surprise me when I am praised for having a remarkable memory, when all I have done is read the label.)

Living in Timothy Dwight was an educational experience in itself. During my first semester, I occupied room 1643, a single room on the first floor. (My brother John had advised me to start out in a single; I could then pick and choose roommates for subsequent semesters.) I once left a formaldehyde-soaked dogfish in the only bathroom on our floor, causing some consternation among my neighbors. The second semester, I shared a room two floors up, with Bill Poindexter, a psychology major from Los Angeles. In my final year, Bill Poindexter and I moved to room 1542, over the building entrance—a magnificent suite. The Yale admissions office assigned us a third roommate, Dick Jennings, a freshman from Clinton, Connecticut, not far from New Haven. His father was a dentist with a practice in Clinton, and the family invited us to their house on several occasions. All three of us became members of Vernon Hall.

Bill Poindexter and I would often take off together on weekends to such places as Wellesley and Smith Colleges and the cities of Washington and New York. He was older than I was, though he looked young (and still does). Whenever we ordered drinks at a bar, he was always asked to produce his draft card. On one occasion Bill hitchhiked to and from Los Angeles for a five-day visit to his home. He packed his clothes in a clean gasoline can that was painted red. He apparently had no difficulty getting rides, the assumption of drivers being that he was trying to get back to a vehicle that had run out of gas—at a time of wartime gasoline rationing.

Many of my classmates in the class of 1945W have remained lifelong friends, among them Mac Gibbons, the late Bill Bliss, and John Finney. I was lucky, too, to befriend Pat Ringling Coerper, of Smith College, and Nickie Passburg, of Wellesley. We exchanged visits on our respective campuses, and I was often invited to their parents' homes. Pat is a descendant of the Ringling circus family and came from Milwaukee; she currently resides in Sarasota, Florida, and has written a history of the Ringling Museum. She has reminded me that she still has my Phi Gam fraternity pin, which I thought I had lost. Nickie came from Longmeadow, Massachusetts, from a family of Danish descent. (Her father was a very successful engineer.) I lost track of Nickie, unfortunately, but I shall never forget a weekend that Bill Poindexter and I spent at Wellesley with her and her roommate. We ended up on Sunday morning renting two canoes at Norumbega Park. In the middle of the lake, Bill got hold of Nickie's paddle and Nickie latched on to Bill's. As each of them tugged the other's paddle, both canoes flipped over. Suddenly, I found myself trying to float, wearing heavy Frank Brothers cordovan shoes. I hurriedly kicked them off to be able to swim to shore. It was an interesting trip back to New Haven, wearing damp clothes and a pair of old borrowed sneakers.

Life in New Haven would have been more difficult without the support of my Aunt Rose, Uncle Haig, and my cousins Dorothy and Nancy. Rose and Haig were more of a father and mother to me than my own parents. Dorothy and Nancy became my "sisters." I always knew that I had a home to go to in Westville and, when they moved from there, at their house in Pine Orchard.

When it came time to choose a medical school, I applied to Yale, Harvard, and Chicago. Applications had to be submitted in the fall of 1944 or early 1945, and at that time most of the spots in the medical schools were destined for members of the navy's V-12 or the army's ASTP programs. Only five or six civilians were accepted in each medical school. I was fortunate to be accepted by all three. Because of my affection for Yale and New Haven and for my aunt's family, I decided to stay at Yale.

I finished my undergraduate program in February, and classes would not start in the Medical School until the fall. Instead of sitting around, I looked for a job as a secondary school science instructor. I visited Saint Paul's School in Concord, New Hampshire, but recognized that arthritis and the very cold, damp weather of New Hampshire would not be a happy combination. Fortunately, I was offered—and accepted—another job, to teach biology, botany, and zoology, at the Irving Preparatory School in Tarrytown, in Westchester County. (The proximity to New York City was appealing.) I had never had much botany except at Victoria College, but the night before I would read what I needed to teach and thus keep just a step ahead of my students. I was very comfortable teaching physics and chemistry. I was a "high school teacher" for just three and a half months but learned a lot from the experience: The school itself was filled with children who were the rejects of New York families. I learned to deal with all sorts of behavior problems. On weekends, I would take off for New York City and beyond, to Smith or Wellesley, much to the chagrin of the headmaster, who felt that masters should stay around on weekends even if they were not on call.

By the time I entered medical school in the fall of 1945, the Second World War was over and we were returning to a four-year course of study (instead of the three-year, round-the-calendar schedule maintained during the war). V-J Day fell just before the opening of the medical school year, and it proved to be a particularly memorable day for me—though not in the way one might expect. I had just moved from Pine Orchard back to New Haven in preparation for the school year and was fortunate to be selected a freshman counselor. The old campus had not yet been renovated, and I was housed in Silliman College, with a first-year law student, Nick Goodspeed from Bridgeport, as my roommate. It being V-J Day, everyone was celebrating. All the restaurants, including all three George and Harry's, were closed, and there was nowhere to get breakfast—or lunch. So I took the old trolley to Branford and was met by Aunt Rose to drive to their beach-front house in Pine Orchard. Pine Orchard was in full celebration. Two houses away there was a magnificent party, where the host offered me an "Orange Blossom." I had no idea that this wonderful, smooth drink consisted of orange juice laid over Scotch whisky. I don't know how many I had or how little I had to eat. However, my next recollection was waking up the following morning on the porch couch at my aunt's house, feeling terrible. I shall never forget V-J Day—or the lesson it taught me about the effects of too much alcohol.

I was glad to start medical school. There were seventy-two of us in the class. Most of the military personnel were released from the armed forces shortly after the beginning of the term, and so all the students were civilians again. It dawned on me that I was surrounded by people who had been in the top one or two of their graduating college classes; the handful of people who came from Yale were certainly tops in their classes (I had ranked second in mine), so we all had to work a lot harder than in undergraduate school.

During the first three years of medical school, I lived on the freshman campus. As a counselor, I was assigned about twenty to twenty-two freshmen and acted as sort of a big brother to them, turning in a report on each of my charges every six weeks. In return for these duties, I received free lodging, some free meals at the Freshman Commons, and a small income. Some of the freshmen coming in after 1945 were war veterans, of course, and considerably older than some of the other students, so there were unusual problems to deal with—for instance, making it clear that a curfew meant a curfew: no female visitors allowed in the dorms after hours.

At Yale Medical School we did not have to take any exams except the first part of the national boards, which came at the end of the second year; if we passed that, we went on to our clinical years. If we did not pass, we had to do something else, or study and take the exam again the following year. We had three months at the end of the second year to study for the exam, and in that time I spent eighteen hours a day studying in my living quarters on the freshman campus across town. Very few students flunked Part 1, but everyone learned who had failed in previous years.

I did my studying in a way that fit my method of learning. Instead of reading a book of histology, a book of pathology, and a book of embryology, I would take an organ such as the kidney and then study its normal anatomy, histology, pathology, and microscopic and gross anatomy, and in that way I cut across the organ systems. If I had picked up a book of histology, I would have been asleep in five minutes. I never got past the first page of the book of embryology because until you get to newborn babies with real embryological defects and resultant diseases, there is no real urgency to know how the gastrointestinal tract rotates in development.

I also learned something about the psychological component in the arthritis I suffered from during this period of my life. For the three months when I was studying for the second-year national boards, I alternated using crutches or a cane, and I managed to get around. After the three mornings and afternoons of the exam, I was having my second beer in the pub around the corner when I realized that I had left my crutches in the exam room. You don't have to work to convince me that there is a psychological layer to every disease.

The chairmanship of surgery at the Yale Medical School changed from the traditional Sam Harvey to the excellent thoracic surgeon Gus Lindskog soon after I arrived. I spent most of my summers subinterning in surgery between the second and third and the third and fourth years. Of course, I didn't know much clinical medicine that first summer, but the other interns and residents were very helpful, and I was exposed to a big dose of clinical medicine.

The Department of Medicine was outstanding, with Dr. Francis Blake as chairman and also as dean of the Medical School. The faculty included Dr. John P. Peters, the renowned chief of metabolism, and Dr. Gerald Klatskin, the hepatologist. As a "clinical clerk" I was responsible for doing a complete initial workup on all patients assigned to me. In addition, in the absence of laboratory technicians available today, I did all the laboratory tests, including urinalysis and blood counts. When I was a third-year student, Dr. Klatskin had a patient with what was then called "catarrhal jaundice" (hepatitis and its virus had not as yet been recognized) in the first room of Fitkin I. One weekend, I was the student on call who had to perform all the blood counts ordered on the ward. Our armamentarium included a cork with a piece of scalpel blade protruding from it to nick the patient's finger and draw a drop of blood. When you had drawn the blood, you wiped the scalpel blade with a piece of gauze soaked in 70 percent alcohol—which (as we now know) does *not* kill viruses. So I went on and stuck all the other patients needing blood counts with the same scalpel. I still have nightmares about how extensively I spread the hepatitis virus. Thank goodness AIDS was not around at that time.

Pediatrics under Dr. Grover Powers was another excellent department. Dr. Powers and his colleague Dr. Dan Darrow attracted many of our classmates to their residency training program. Microbiology and immunology had no stars, but the faculty were dedicated teachers of the entire spectrum, including parasitology. Dr. Treffers, one of my thesis advisors, taught us the basics of immunology, including the emerging field of tissue immunology that involved my thesis work in multiple sclerosis.

Obstetrics and gynecology was not on a par with the other departments. The chair was Dr. Toms, whose claim to fame was the development of pelvimetry to measure radiographically the potential of the maternal pelvis to accommodate the passage of the fetal head at birth. It was a way to select some candidates for cesarean section. Lying-in and natural childbirth had just come in. I delivered or assisted in the delivery of sixteen babies; I was scared to death and never quite sure of what was happening. My salvation was the good supervision available and the knowledge that babies have been born for thousands of years without much help.

The most shocking experience I had was assisting in one cesarean section. It was a Saturday night, and a big Medical School dance was scheduled. We drew straws to see who would skip the dance to stay on call. I lost. Around 7:00 P.M. I got a call that we were going to do a cesarean section on a private patient. The "dean" of obstetricians for New Haven society was going to deliver one of the community's young matrons. As was customary, the intern and I started our ten-minute scrub with antiseptic soap ahead of the resident and the senior obstetrician. Shortly thereafter, the senior resident joined us. Eventually the obstetrician arrived. His scrub lasted a little over a minute, rather than the mandatory ten. To go from the washroom into the operating room you were trained to use your derrière. He pushed the door open with his wet hand. The scrub nurse assisted him with his sterile gown and gloves. He immediately put his hand up to adjust the operating room light—this was in 1949, a time when there were no sterile handles—thus contaminating his gloves. After the senior resident put the sterile drapes over the patient's abdomen, the surgeon picked up the scalpel and with one stroke cut through the skin, the muscle, the peritoneum, and the enlarged uterus. Blood was gushing all over. The senior resident and intern were clamping bleeders as fast as possible and finally got the situation under control. Fortunately, the baby was unhurt and healthy. The obstetrician left immediately thereafter. The senior resident, the intern, and I sewed everything back up. The patient had an uneventful recovery. It should be emphasized that 1949 was still in the early era of antibiotics or substantial blood transfusion.

In the dressing room after the operation I asked the senior resident why that obstetrician was allowed to operate. His response was that they always scrubbed in a senior resident to bail him out. Also he was held in the highest regard by the upper crust of New Haven society. It was a lesson I have never forgotten; I was lucky to have missed the dance. In all my years of surgery, I never tolerated such incompetent surgeons, nor would I subscribe to using senior residents "to bail out" unqualified faculty. Today, peer review and the guidelines for accreditation are such that incompetent physicians can be identified quickly.

Quite early on in medical school, we had to decide on a thesis, which was required to graduate. Most students were in a laboratory by the end of the second year, and Yale provided us with a little money to do some sort of research. Some students waited almost until the last minute and then just found some clinical cases of this or that and wrote them up as a clinical study. Yale was pretty lenient about it, and I am not aware that any-one in my time had been denied graduation because of a poor thesis. My own thesis was in two related parts, one clinical and one experimental. I was interested in the origins of multiple sclerosis, in part because one of my mentors was Bill German, the professor of neurosurgery, who had his specialty boards in neurology as well as neurosurgery. Yale had neither a separate division of neurology nor even a separate professor of neurology. Dr. German would see all the multiple sclerosis patients coming to the Yale New Haven Hospital, and I worked with him for three years. At that time, there were two prevalent theories about the cause of MS. One was that of Dr. Tracy Putnam, of Columbia University Neurological Institute in New York, who proposed that venular thromboses of the brain lead to the patchy degeneration of the white matter. The other theory was that MS was an autoimmune disease whereby patients produced antibodies destructive to their own brain tissue. Following Dr. Putnam's theory, we treated patients with anticoagulants, heparin, and dicoumerol. That is how I learned the use of anticoagulants, a knowledge that I brought to Duke and applied to thrombotic disorders. Nobody at Duke at that time had ever used that combination of drugs.

In my laboratory research, I worked with Dr. Treffers, the professor of immunology. I took guinea pigs, immunized them to their own white brain substance, and tried to see if we could develop what was called "iso-allergic demyelinization." The Medical School supplied us with money to buy the guinea pigs. Just around the corner from my lab was the division of experimental pathology, where the famous Dr. Harry Greene, who headed the division of surgical pathology, used to implant tumors in guinea pigs' eyes to study them histologically. He offered me some one-eyed guinea pigs at a discount, so I wouldn't have to go to the farm to pick up fresh guinea pigs. I told him that one-eyed guinea pigs in which he had implanted tumors probably had compromised immune systems and wouldn't be suitable for our experiments. He then sent me to a guinea pig farm near Waterbury where I paid two or three times the price for my guinea pigs. Years later, I discovered that Dr. Greene also owned the guinea pig farm, so he had a monopoly on the animals.

One day Dr. Greene came to the room in which eight of us studied microscopic pathology. He was to be our instructor for the day. When he came in, he asked what was the subject for the day; we said it was glomerulonephritis. He said, "Nobody really knows a damn about that form of kidney disease," and stomped out.

There were other memorable instructors at that time, people whom I consider mentors. Dr. William Gardner, the chairman of anatomy, was a wonderful teacher. He was an endocrinologist, as were most members of the Anatomy Department at Yale. Dr. Gardner looked very young. When I first met him, the day before the start of medical school, I was walking around the gross anatomy laboratory, looking for a female cadaver. I had been told to try to get a female, since they were quite rare compared to the larger collection of male cadavers. Dr. Gardner walked in to the laboratory and without introducing himself said, "Can I help you?" I thought he was a laboratory assistant of some type and told him frankly that I was looking for the table numbers of the few female cadavers. He smiled and walked away. You can imagine how I felt the next day, sitting in the front row of the anatomy lecture room, when "the professor of anatomy" walked in. He looked at me and smiled, and never in our many subsequent years of friendship did he bring up the subject of our first encounter. As it turned out, my cadaver mate, "Bud" (Dewitt) Baldwin, and I ended up with a female cadaver. There was really not that big a difference.

One further lesson I learned from Bill Gardner was to tear up your lecture notes each semester so as to stay fresh with the subject material. For many decades I followed his example.

Another minor character in the Anatomy Department was Professor Harold Burr, the head of the Division of Neuroanatomy. He never used notes, and he drew pictures of the brain and spinal cord with chalk on the blackboard simultaneously with both hands. He made his lectures interesting by correlating the anatomy with specific lesions of brain and cord disorders. For example, the anatomy of the spinal cord became more salient when we were learning the site of degeneration in amyotrophic lateral sclerosis—better known as Lou Gehrig's disease.

Perhaps the best department in the basic sciences was pathology. Our first-year courses correlated basic science with instruction about disease, that is, integrating normal and abnormal histology. The chairman, Dr. Milton Winternitz, had been a distinguished faculty member at Johns Hopkins before coming to Yale. Before World War II he had been the dean of the Yale Medical School and had built up an excellent pathology faculty, dedicated, as he was, to teaching. Every member of the faculty came to the lectures given by other members of the faculty and sat quietly in the back row. I presume they were the peer review group for the lecture presentations.

Dr. Winternitz lived on Prospect Hill, near the Yale chemistry laboratory. Each morning at 7:30 A.M., wearing a soft hat and with his hands clasped behind his back, he would walk across the Yale campus, past the freshman campus, where I would join him on his path, either just in front of him or a few steps behind, for the rest of our walk across town to the Medical School. Never did we exchange a single word.

Dr. Winternitz was about five feet one inch tall, but he was a tiger. He knew every student: he had studied each one by picture and background before he gave the roll call the first day. The day you showed up, he had a nickname picked for you, and mine—"Phenylalanine"—was one of the more polite ones. It was Dr. Winternitz who, at the conclusion of one of our gross pathology demonstration classes, stood at the laboratory door and punched every student coming out in the solar plexus—including me, in my duraluminum brace. He had his revenge, though, in a subsequent gross pathology class, when he asked me to lower the venetian blinds because of the sun's glare. I couldn't get the blinds down, and they became all tangled up. He then said in front of the whole class, "Phenylalanine, you wouldn't even be a good domestic."

One student pushed familiarity too far by calling him Winter—the name his senior colleagues used for him and that we used behind his back. Dr. Winternitz put his arm around the student and suggested sarcastically, "Why don't you call me Miltie?"

Despite such incidents, Dr. Winternitz was admired for his distinguished academic achievement, his commitment to teaching, and his chairmanship. We felt lucky to have had him as our professor before he retired, and held it an honor to have been his student. When it came to dedicating our senior class show, which was the first of its kind, our honoree was Dr. Winternitz. When I became dean of the Duke Medical School, one of my models for quality in department heads was Dr. Winternitz; the primary purpose of a department in the Medical School is always teaching, even if other functions generate more income.

Pharmacology was a bit of a joke. Dr. Salter, a specialist in thyroid metabolism, was the chairman, and one of the songs in our senior class play was entitled "Dr. Salter, Dr. Salter—when do we learn pharmacology?" One unforgettable laboratory demonstration was on alcohol and coordination. The lecturer, at the beginning of his discussion, asked for four volunteers. The first was to receive a placebo dose of alcohol containing zero alcohol but smelling like a real drink. Number 2 would receive the same volume of a drink with one ounce of alcohol. Number 3 would get two ounces, and number 4 would receive three ounces. All four underwent manual coordination exercises in front of the whole class before taking their assigned aliquot. Thirty minutes later they were retested. What had not been evaluated beforehand was that the classmate who received no alcohol had never had a drink thereof. He was the classic picture of a drunk—his coordination was way off. The classmate who got the three ounces was a heavy drinker, and his coordination improved 100 percent. Somehow the results were leaked to the *Yale Daily News*. The ensuing headlines stated, "Yale pharmacology professor shows alcohol improves coordination." As I recall, the professor left Yale shortly thereafter.

Four years earlier, the Pharmacology Department had lost two of its better faculty—the principal authors of the standard pharmacology textbook, Louis Goodman and Alfred Gilman, who had both been at Yale during my brother John's student days. However, Yale allowed you to structure your own way of learning, and we were able to make up some of the deficit on our own, which in my case was by reading.

By the time I graduated from medical school, I was married and had an infant son (see chapter 16). I had spent five and a half years at Yale and thought that for my internship I needed to see a different part of the country. I knew that I liked academic medicine because my thesis work led me to believe that I enjoyed research, so I was pointed toward an academic career in surgery. I was chatting one day with the chief resident in neurosurgery, who happened to have interned at Duke, and he asked me whether I had thought of Duke. I said I didn't think I'd even heard of Duke and I didn't know where it was. He described it, and I applied.

My relationship with Yale did not end upon graduation. In addition to maintaining my status as a loyal alumnus of both the undergraduate school and the Medical School (attending with great pleasure my fiftieth

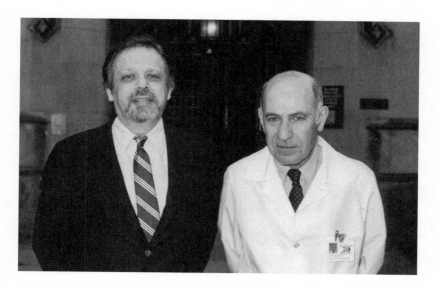

3   President Bart Giamatti of Yale University visiting
the Duke campus, 1972. DUMC Photography.

and fifty-fifth 1945W undergraduate class reunions and my fiftieth 1949
Medical School reunion), I have maintained the connections in various
ways.

While he was president of Yale, Dr. Bart Giamatti visited me at Duke,
and in our talk together, I took advantage of his expertise as an historian. We discussed the role of private philanthropy, Christianity, and the
founding of private universities. I was preparing a major speech on the history of Harvard, Yale, Princeton, Johns Hopkins, Duke, Chicago and Stanford, a range that I addressed on more than one occasion, though never to
great applause. He was gentle, kind, and understanding. When Giamatti
was later in the midst of tough union negotiations at Yale, I worried how
such a modest humanist would fare, just as I did when Douglas Maitland
Knight, another Yale humanist, was president of Duke and dealing with
union problems.

When Dr. Benno Schmidt later became president of Yale, he invited
me to serve on the President's Council and to serve as the council's chairman on the Medical Center. He also gave me the opportunity to propose
the membership of my committee, which included Dr. Frederick Battaglia
of the Department of Pediatrics, University of Colorado Health Sciences

Center, Denver; John W. Colloton, CEO of the University of Iowa Hospitals; Dr. Philip Leder, Department of Genetics, Harvard Medical School; Dr. Robert G. Petersdorf, president, Association of American Medical Colleges; and Dr. Virginia V. Weldon, vice president of scientific affairs, Monsanto Company. For five years the committee met twice a year. For the first three years we reported to Benno. For the next two years we reported to Dr. Richard (Rick) Levin, who had been named Benno's successor. Our committee was immensely pleased that Rick picked up on all our recommendations to Benno and implemented most of them.

In recent years, I have been pleased to see the evolution of Yale under President Levin. The renaissance of the physical plant now under way was long overdue. It is now a source of pride to visit the campus. Even though Duke University has been my home and charge for over fifty years, I have not lost my interest and regard for my alma mater.

3

I WAS ASKED TO start my surgical internship a week early, on June 23, 1949, to relieve a graduating intern going to another institution. To do so, I felt it prudent to skip the graduation exercises at Yale and get settled in Durham before starting work at Duke. My graduation consisted of having a beer with my brother John in New Haven while putting an M.D. caduceus on the rear license plate of my little Plymouth. John, who was by then board-certified in general and thoracic surgery, was moving back to Yale to become an instructor in the Department of Surgery, and he and his wife, Betty, took over our New Haven garden apartment, at Green Gardens Court in East Haven.

In Durham, as in New Haven, apartments were hard to find; the influx of house officers coming back from the armed services for graduate training, combined with the lack of construction during the war years, had created a major housing shortage. But we had the help of some good friends of my wife's brother-in-law, Julian Brantley. Roy Parker—who was completing his training in ob-gyn at Duke and who had been Julian's undergraduate classmate at the University of North Carolina—and his wife, Georgia, found us a small one-bedroom apartment in the Kimbro Apartments, located in the woods within walking distance of Duke Hospital.

Durham in the late forties was still rural, better known as a mill and tobacco town than as the "City of Medicine" it is today. Coming into town, my wife and I drove down Erwin Road, a two-lane road ending at what is now Trent Drive. The only building there was the one later called the Hanes Annex (recently renamed for Dr. John Hope Franklin), and at that point Erwin Road became a winding one-lane road through the beginning of the eight-thousand-acre Duke Forest. Erwin Road is now a busy four lanes, and there is no vestige of the forest nearby.

The Kimbro Apartments were a new speculative venture built next to the Dutch Village Motel on Elba Street, an unpaved road rich in chicken coops. A one-bedroom apartment went for eighty-five a month. Further up the road were small shacks where weekend celebrations often featured the sounds of gunshots and police sirens.

We found our apartment, 1B, but no furniture—that arrived ten days later. Our new neighbors, many of them fellow house staff members, were both hospitable and generous. They loaned us a mattress, sheets, towels, and cooking utensils; in short, the basics for everyday life. It was hot as Hades, so a little rubber fan was one of our first purchases from Sawyer & Moore, the drugstore on Main Street.

My income at that time consisted of a monthly allowance of $225 from my father and an anticipated monthly wage of $12.50 from Duke because I was married. Single house officers received no pay. White uniforms were furnished by the hospital, and uniform laundry was gratis. Our meals at the hospital were also free and most commonly featured pork chops; on weekends we could invite our spouses and our children for dinner.

It was a ten-minute walk to Duke hospital from the Kimbro Apartments. There was a shortcut through the woods, going past a row of cabins where the unmarried male house staff lived, but the disadvantage of this route was that it tended to mess up one's clean, starched white uniforms.

Despite the fact that it had existed for only nineteen years, the Duke Medical School and its accompanying hospital impressed me as being a very mature organization. It had been founded by the generosity of James Buchanan Duke, whose fortune was based on the tobacco and electric power industries. A native of Durham, Mr. Duke recognized that the area lagged well behind the rest of the nation in the provision of health care as well as in the educational opportunities offered its citizens. He set about correcting these deficiencies. By his indenture of 1924 he provided, among other things, for a four-year medical school and a four-hundred-bed hospital as part of a major expansion of Trinity College; two generations of the Duke family had been generous benefactors of the college, a fine small liberal arts school, since its founding in 1836. James B. Duke's magnificent gift enabled President Few to achieve his and Mr. Duke's ultimate dream: to create a major new university with a graduate school as well as professional schools.

Wilburt Cornell Davison was brought in as the first head of Duke's medical school and hospital. He had been educated at Princeton and Oxford, working with the great Sir William Osler, and had then trained as a pediatrician at Johns Hopkins. Dr. Davison attracted to Duke an outstanding, primarily young faculty—many from Hopkins, the institution that served as the model for Duke's medical enterprise.

The doors of the Duke hospital and the medical school opened in the depths of the Depression, and it quickly became apparent that there was not enough money to pay the clinical faculty their full salaries. At that time a professor of surgery might have earned $5,000 a year, yet through the university's endowment Dr. Davison could afford to pay only half of that. Deryl Hart, the chairman of surgery, suggested that they make up the other $2,500 from the pooled income from the clinical practice. Davison agreed, and right away clinical practice assumed a very important role at Duke, at a time when clinical work, other than on a consultant basis, was frowned upon in academic medical circles. At Hopkins, for example, full-time faculty did not have ongoing patient care responsibilities, so they could concentrate on their teaching and do some research, although most clinicians did not do the kind of research we see today. Interestingly, during the years I was head of the Medical Center, the financial contribution from the university never increased: from 1930 to 1989, $2,500 is all the university ever contributed to the salary of a clinical faculty member. From 1964 on, however, many other medical schools recognized the importance of Duke's group practice mechanism and adopted it.

Back in 1930–32, Davison and Hart were worried that the referring physicians in North Carolina would view Duke's group practice as a competitive threat, so they applied the term "private diagnostic clinic" (PDC) to describe it. The implication—and the fact—was that patients sent to Duke for diagnosis would then be sent back to their referring physicians for treatment.

Early on, Dr. Davison established an arm's-length relationship between the PDCs and the hospital. The PDCs (one surgical and one medical) were to be run by the chairmen of the clinical departments, especially Deryl Hart, chairman of surgery, and Eugene Stead, chairman of medicine. Dr. Davison left the responsibility for the PDCs entirely to them. Except for sponsoring the graduation dinner of the senior class, I know of no other contribution that the clinical departments made to the day-to-day operations of the hospital. The departments did contribute to the building fund, as it has been known, contributing 4 percent of their gross earnings (subsequently 8 percent) to a construction fund that helped finance the evolution and construction of more and better clinical facilities, generally in proportion to the fiscal contribution of the department. When an addition to the hospital was built in 1957, for instance, the departments of medicine and surgery got the largest share, and pediatrics, which had contributed very little to the building fund, got little.

After World War II, the National Institutes of Health (NIH) came into being, and research funding grew exponentially. Research became a very big enterprise at Duke, as elsewhere. So in the fifties, Dr. Davison realized that he headed more than just a medical school, more than just a hospital and clinics, more than just a research institute. That is when the term "Duke Medical Center" came into use.

Duke is fortunate in having its medical school and hospital both under one corporate roof. At Yale, there is the medical school and a separate corporation for Yale–New Haven Hospital; at Harvard, there is the medical school and a plethora of independent hospitals. Duke, from the beginning, had a strong basis for centralization.

By 1949 the Duke Medical Center buzzed with activity eighteen to twenty hours a day. There were no empty wings of buildings, such as one saw in New Haven; every cubic inch was used. Dr. Davison did not meet me at the front door on my first day; it would be several weeks before I had the privilege of meeting him. But his presence permeated the entire institution—I could feel it.

My first rotation, lasting through the end of June, was on Dr. Hart's private general surgical service. The day before I began the rotation, a Saturday, I made rounds on all the patients I would inherit from the departing intern. Early on Sunday morning, I rounded again with Bill Shingleton, the senior surgical resident on Dr. Hart's service. At 9 A.M. I was paged to report to Dr. Hart's office on the third floor to start rounds with him. Unfortunately, I zigged instead of zagged and ended up walking from Cabell Ward, the private surgical ward, through the double-door entrance to Meyer Ward, the closed psychiatric unit. Once you entered through the first door of Meyer, you were locked in unless you had the key, which I did not. To make matters worse, in the absence of air-conditioning, there was a large, noisy fan on the first door. Realizing I was trapped, and that my chief was waiting for our initial meeting, I started pounding on the door. Nobody paid any attention. After a painful ten minutes, a nurse with a key finally came. I never knew how Dr. Hart received my explanation, but I assume he had heard that excuse before.

During my first week, Dr. Hart, with Bill Shingleton as first assistant, removed the diseased gallbladder of a fifty-five-year-old man. As second assistant, I stood next to Dr. Hart, holding retractors for maximum exposure. In the recovery room the patient showed signs of significant bleeding, and we had to take him back to the operating room to find the cause and to stop the bleeding. On reexploration, we found that the abdomen was filled with blood and blood clots. Dr. Hart soaked a succession of large surgical pads with the blood and dropped them to the floor on my only pair of white bucks (twenty-six dollars at Frank Brothers in New Haven). Given the tense situation and my very junior status, I didn't utter a peep. The bleeding was controlled, the patient was saved, and thereafter I always kept a pair of old red-brown shoes in the OR locker to wear when I was to scrub.

The interns worked in pairs on the various services, and we worked every other night. On some services, like general surgery, you didn't leave on your night off until your work on your own ward was completed. On other services, like neurosurgery, you left about 5:30 P.M. after afternoon rounds, because generally you had been up the night before taking care of the very sick postoperative patients of the day. When that happened, I would go home and promptly fall asleep on the sofa. From the point of view of physical demands, it was tough sledding for the interns. But my internship year was one of the two years in my life when I learned more than I did at any other times in my life: my internship year, because that is when I really got into the trenches and was responsible for patients, and my chief residency year, when I had ultimate responsibility.

The residency system at Duke was not a pyramidal system where twelve people would enter and only one would become chief resident; it was more of a blunted pyramid, a block system. It was hierarchic, so that the intern was supervised by the junior assistant resident, who was supervised in turn by the senior assistant resident, and the senior assistant resident by the chief resident. On each service, faculty supervised the resident staff. On general surgery, Dr. Clarence Gardner kept an appropriately close eye on the residency. Residents were free to call in anybody from the faculty or from another service to consult at any time. On neurosurgery, Dr. Barnes Woodhall or Dr. Guy Odom was with us at all times, whether we were seeing a private or public patient. (Duke Hospital since its inception had assumed the responsibility to serve the sick and poor of the community, and the term "public patient" refers to a patient receiving free care.)

The week spent on Dr. Hart's service gave me a quick introduction to the surgical service, so that by July 1, when I moved to neurosurgery, I was no longer a total tenderfoot. Barnes Woodhall and Guy Odom, the chief and senior neurosurgeon respectively, had international reputations. Dr. Woodhall had been trained by Dr. Walter Dandy at Johns Hopkins. A master surgeon who never wasted a motion, Dr. Woodhall was a Yankee from Maine and still had some of the characteristics of a no-nonsense operator. Dr. Odom was a native of New Orleans who had trained under Dr. Wilder Penfield at the Montreal Neurological Institute. At first I thought he spoke with a Brooklyn accent, but it turned out to be New Orleans English. The two men had great mutual respect for each other. Their personalities, styles of operating, and interests were different but complementary: Dr. Woodhall was interested in the vascular components of the brain and aneurysms, while Dr. Odom studied brain tumors and neuropathology. I would have been comfortable if either one had operated on my family or me.

On my first day on their service, I was shocked to see the operative schedule for neurosurgery for the day, all to take place in the same room. At least two brain tumors were scheduled, with diagnostic air studies preceding each, as well as a few lesser neurosurgical operations such as the removal of ruptured intervertebral discs and peripheral nerve repairs. In New Haven, it was a big day when a single craniotomy for a brain tumor was scheduled with the preceding diagnostic air studies—the craniotomy would last six to eight hours, since Dr. Harvey Cushing's tedious dissection techniques were used. Drs. Woodhall and Odom rarely took more than three hours to do a craniotomy. Dr. Woodhall used the Dandy finger dissection method to remove large bulky tumors. The first such operation I witnessed made me wonder if he had lost his mind, but the patients did better with a much shorter operation.

The quality of care on neurosurgery was immaculate, and the training was rigorous and thorough. Rounds with the residents would start at 6:30 A.M. Afternoon rounds on multiple wards began at 4 P.M. and ended at 5:30 P.M. If you were on call, you worked up the new patients and made rounds again at 9 P.M. You woke up at 2 A.M. to round again on the fresh postoperative cases.

The three major figures in general surgery at the time were Dr. Deryl Hart, Dr. Clarence Gardner, and Dr. Keith Grimson. Dr. Hart had many research interests. One was the use of ultraviolet lights to control infections in the intraoperative period in the operating room. This did not receive much national attention, but many people at Duke were convinced that it kept down the transmission of infections at a time when we did not have laminar air flow and other methods in use today to prevent staphylococcal infections in the operating room. Dr. Hart had also done some research on hamsters to determine whether pregnancy early or late in the ovulatory cycle produced males or females. He had also done some work on empyemas, pockets of infection in the chest, before I came to Duke. By any standard he was a master clinical surgeon. Almost by instinct he tended to make all the correct surgical decisions. We learned by observation rather than sets of rules.

On the Wednesday night before each Thanksgiving, Dr. Hart and his wife, Mary, invited all the residents and interns in general and thoracic surgery for a turkey dinner at their beautiful home. Mary knew the backgrounds of the interns and their spouses, the names of all their children and what illnesses they had recently had. She and Deryl formed a team that served Duke well when he was chairman of the Department of Surgery and subsequently when he became president of Duke University from 1960 to 1963.

Dr. Gardner was a classical general surgeon who taught us the fundamentals of surgery. He operated by the textbook, in contrast to Dr. Hart, who was a genius at improvisation and at using new and different approaches. As a teacher, Dr. Gardner did not tolerate mediocrity or uncertainty: either you felt an enlarged spleen or you did not—vague answers were not accepted.

Both Hart and Gardner had been trained in the meticulous Hopkins tradition established by Dr. William Halsted. Dr. Grimson had not: he came from the University of Chicago, and sometimes his different approach led to problems. He used catgut instead of silk. He was particularly interested in doing total sympathectomies for hypertension (this was the era before antihypertensive drugs) and vagotomies for peptic ulcers and was a pioneer in peripheral vascular surgery. He had an active research program in these fields and was a leader in clinical pharmacology. He had about the only clinical research laboratory at Duke at the time, and he let Bill Shingleton and me use his fluoroscopic facilities, both for patients and for the dogs that we used as experimental subjects.

Each of these surgeons took turns with student rounds. Dr. Gardner ran the surgical outpatient clinic, where he had a class every afternoon in which two or three of the most interesting patients were presented. It was a wonderful educational exercise for me, as an intern, to sneak in there and listen to these presentations. Dr. Hart, by contrast, worked best one-on-one. His main function, as I saw it as a house officer, was to represent the Department of Surgery at meetings with Dr. Davison and the other chairmen. He also represented Duke on the national scene. He was ultimately in charge of the educational program in surgery, although Dr. Gardner also played a significant role.

Dr. Hart had a great deal of discretionary power in dealing with members of the department, especially in allocating salaries, but he was scrupulously fair. At the end of the year Dr. Hart would see what the earnings of the group practice were, and he would look at the productivity of each faculty member, not just in terms of how many patients each one saw but also how much he or she contributed to the academic stature of the department. Then he would call us in one by one and tell us what he thought our salary ought to be. As far as I know, only one person ever challenged him on salary, and it was not me. Hart's reputation for fairness was part of the reason he was eventually appointed president of Duke University, at a time of some turmoil for the institution.

Dr. Lenox Baker was a legend in orthopedic surgery. He was a taskmaster who could be rather stern with the house staff, though he was thoroughly respected by everyone. On my first day as his intern, his chief resident, Dr. Leonard Goldner, gave me the advice to "just smile and laugh if he gets on your back." It worked. To Dr. Baker's credit, he established a broad, multihospital orthopedic residency program. He not only trained a generation of orthopedic surgeons but also provided a network of visiting clinics in North Carolina. These clinics have been a source of referrals to other services at Duke as well as orthopedics.

Urology was blessed with faculty who excelled in their clinical work. They were led by Dr. Ed Alyea and Dr. John Dees, both trained at Johns Hopkins. The two men got on well with each other and were respected by all their colleagues, although their personalities and professional and extracurricular interests differed. In later years, I got to know them better— Dr. Alyea and his love for fishing off the shores of his house at Kerr Lake and Dr. Dees during the hunting season. Dees was something of an innovator, and he developed a technique to make a coagulant pull out stones from the kidney. John's wife, Dr. Susan Dees, was equally well known for her work in pediatric allergy and immunology.

I had a rather embarrassing incident involving Dr. Alyea. At Christmastime during my internship year, I received a package of unknown origin that contained a beautiful and delicious baked ham. Not until the last ounce was consumed did I notice that the addressee was Alyea, not Anlyan. I confessed to him, fully expecting a reprimand. Instead he laughed and said he hoped that we had enjoyed it.

After the founding chief of thoracic surgery, Dr. Josiah Trent, died tragically young in December 1948, Dr. Will Sealy was appointed to succeed him. He was just returning from special training at the University of Michigan when I started at Duke. In 1949 pulmonary tuberculosis was the predominant disease requiring surgical intervention. It would take Sealy a number of years to develop a first-rate program in thoracic surgery, through appointments of such talented people as Dr. Glenn Young and Dr. Ivan Brown, who evolved open-heart surgery.

In the late 1940s interns spent six weeks working in the blood bank. At 9 P.M. on the night before I began this rotation, just as I was on my way home to get some sleep, I ran into Ivan Brown, who headed the service. I did not leave until 2 A.M., after getting a thorough indoctrination in crossmatching and blood banking. Brown had developed and operated the laboratories of the 65th General Hospital, Duke's unit in England during World War II. In the years that followed, he rejoined Duke's surgical residency program to finish his training. We ended up as co-residents in general and thoracic surgery.

Dr. Kenneth L. Pickrell was an excellent technical surgeon in plastic and reconstructive surgery. Through some quirk, I did not get a rotation through plastic surgery; however, I have long admired the training program he established, which has included many plastic surgeons who trained under him and under his successor, Dr. Nicholas G. Georgiade, who was a surgical intern along with me in January 1950.

When I came to Duke, there was a combined eye, ear, nose, and throat residency in the Department of Surgery. Dr. Banks Anderson was a first-rate clinical ophthalmologist and probably the most laconic individual I have ever met. You could rarely get him to tell you what was wrong. Dr. Watt Eagle and Dr. Ralph Arnold ran the ENT side. Dr. Eagle was a bon vivant who had trained at Hopkins, and he spent most of the time doing tonsillectomies and adenoidectomies. Occasionally he would take out a styloid process for intractable headaches; I doubt that this is seen today as a very good operation, but it was typical of ear, nose, and throat specialists in that era. They were so busy with tonsillectomies that they really didn't open any other major avenues of activity or study. When the new antibiotics came into being and slashed the high rate of tonsillectomies, ENT doctors started looking for other areas to develop.

Dr. Joe Beard, who headed the division of experimental surgery, was

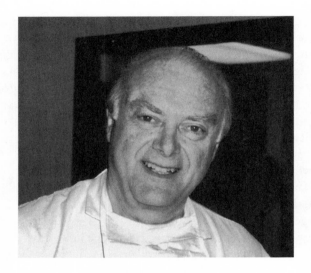

4   A devoted friend and longtime associate, Dr. Nicholas G. Georgiade, pro-
fessor and chief of plastic surgery. Dr. Georgiade was a fellow surgical intern of
Dr. Anlyan's in 1950 and a close faculty colleague until his death in 2001. DUMC
Photography.

one of the more delightful characters on our faculty in the mid-century.
Dr. Beard was trained as a surgeon, but while he was at Vanderbilt and at
Rockefeller University—then known as the Rockefeller Institute—he became fascinated by tumor virology. He and his wife, Dorothy Beard, devoted their lives to the study of viruses that might cause cancer. Dr. Beard
is usually remembered for developing a vaccine to cure sleeping sickness in
horses. The royalties from that vaccine contributed to the start in 1947 of
the Bell Building, the Medical Center's first research building. Dr. Beard
also did important work on avian tumor viruses. In 1952 he gave a talk
to the Society of University Surgeons when the group met at Duke. He
showed what he thought were virus particles of avian leukosis by electron
microscopy, and he brought down the house when he said he didn't know
if what he was showing was the virus or some of his dandruff.

The Beards were familiar to all the medical students because in the second year of the curriculum they taught surgery using dogs. Sometime at
the end of the fifties, they got tired of teaching dog surgery and convinced
Dr. Hart to turn the responsibility over to me. I was apprehensive that the
Beards might be somewhat resentful of a young whippersnapper coming

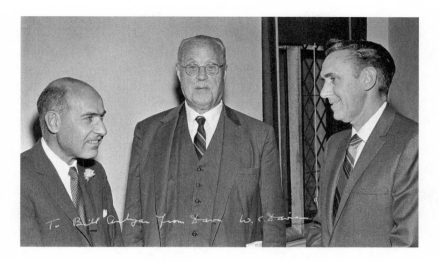

5   Dr. W. G. Anlyan greeting the founding dean, Dr. Wilburt C. Davison, and alumnus Dr. John Yarborough of Maryville, Tennessee. DUMC Photography.

in and changing the course considerably, as I planned to do. But they were very supportive. I had become the Medical Education for National Defense (MEND) coordinator, a new post at many medical schools, and so my objective was not to teach a student how to take out the spleen or the appendix of a dog, but instead to look at the vast problems we would have if there were mass casualties after an atomic attack. I had been briefed in this regard by a special course at Walter Reed Medical Center in 1956. The basic philosophy was that you dealt only with those you could save, but not the severely injured because they would take up too much time in a mass casualty situation. We needed to teach students how to perform life-saving measures such as tracheotomies and tube thoracotomies, procedures that were simple to do and that would save a patient's life, instead of trying to save a person who had fifty holes in the intestines and feces all over and who was almost certainly past saving.

Finally, there was the legendary Dr. Wilburt Cornell Davison. Early in my internship, I encountered him in the hallway by accident. Meeting this tall, fairly heavy, very outgoing man who had created the Medical School and built the hospital was a special occasion. Once you met him, he left you with the feeling that he had known you for some time. He knew my background and never forgot to send me a postcard from Cairo when he visited there. On one occasion I received such a card in the morning and met him in the dining room at lunchtime. The wonders of air travel, even in 1950!

Drs. Davison, Hart, and Grimson all had summer homes in Roaring Gap, in the mountains of North Carolina. Dr. Hart vacationed during August; Dr. Grimson took long weekends during the summer; and Dr. Davison was in and out, not only in the mountains but throughout the world. (One of Dr. Davison's achievements was to select medical students in their senior year who would serve as primary care physicians in Roaring Gap.)

By 1940 Dr. Davison had become an important figure on the national and international health scenes. He was on many important national committees and worked closely with the Department of Defense as well as the Veterans Administration. As a result of his peripatetic life style, between 1950 and 1960 the affairs of the Medical School appeared to be mainly in the hands of an oligarchy of department chairmen. Dr. Philip Handler, chairman of biochemistry, was the leader of the basic sciences group, while Dr. Deryl Hart and Dr. Eugene Stead, chairman of the Department of Medicine, led the clinical departments. These men were not necessarily in concert on major policy matters; but they were counterbalancing forces, each cognizant that the number 1 rule was to do what was best for the university, its Medical School, and the teaching hospital.

One of the things that impressed me about Dr. Eugene Stead, as well as many of the very senior ob-gyn people such as Drs. Nick Carter, Buck Thomas, and Bob Creadick, was that when I finished my residency in 1955 and had what I would call the "left-over practice" of the surgical PDC, they referred their private patients for general surgical consultation directly to me. I was touched that, although they obviously had access to all the most senior people in the surgical service, they would help out the young man who was coming along. If Dr. Stead referred an emergency patient who needed to have an operation in the middle of the night, he would spend the night standing behind me in the operating room, watching what went on. This always reminded me of the attention given to cases by Sir William Osler, who, when he was chairman of medicine at Hopkins, used to take his students and residents on rounds to the autopsy room to see why the patient had died.

For some reason, possibly because we sometimes discussed how things could be improved, Dr. Hart asked me to help him with some administrative problems. A few of them, such as the operation of the emergency room, got me in trouble in the early years of my residency, particularly with the

Department of Medicine, which was very competitive for patients coming through the emergency room. But one success led to another request, and by the time I finished the residency program, Dr. Hart had essentially put me in charge of recruiting interns and residents and working out the rotations.

In the case of the emergency room, I wanted the surgical service to have more authority to deal with patients, because the assignments were made by the nurse in charge, and sometimes patients who needed attention from other services should have been seen more promptly. Sam Martin, who was in charge of the clinics and the emergency room for the Department of Medicine at the time, was miffed that I suggested more control by the surgical service. But I prevailed.

Up to that time, the whole internship recruitment process had been improvised out of the pockets of Dr. Hart and Dr. Gardner. When Dr. Hart turned it over to me, Dr. Gardner was very happy to get rid of the responsibility. I changed the process by introducing a set way in which applicants were invited to visit us and then established a formal schedule of tours, faculty interviews, and subsequent compilation of the data on each applicant. In essence we formalized the application process before the current system, the national matching program, was in place, in which prospective interns send their applications to a central clearing house in Washington. We got much better applicants and more from other institutions. Until that time, we had had a preponderance of Duke graduates. I also paid more attention to the rotations the interns would have and what their preferences were, whereas previously that duty had been assigned to the upcoming chief resident for the year. This way there was a continuity of responsibility for the interns' education.

Somewhat to my surprise, I also started doing a research project at Duke early in my residency. Having done some research on the use of anticoagulants to treat multiple sclerosis as part of my Yale thesis, I considered research an important part of my career. Duke interns were not supposed to be doing research, but it became obvious that there was no one else who knew how to use heparin and dicumerol as anticoagulants in thrombotic diseases of the veins and arteries. I do not believe that I made any great advances in the understanding of multiple sclerosis. (Its exact cause is still a mystery.) However, my involvement with that disease under Dr. Bill German at Yale was what set the stage for my entry into the field of thrombotic disorders during my internship at Duke.

During my residency I was asked to see every patient at Duke Hospital who had deep-venous thrombosis or some thrombotic disorder on the arterial side and who might be a candidate for the administration of an anticoagulant. In the course of a very short time, I became a major consultant in managing coagulation disorders of patients on most services at Duke and developed a team of younger residents in surgery who worked with me. At one point, I calculated that we had treated over seven hundred patients.

I received my first NIH grant at the beginning of my junior assistant residency, that is, my second year at Duke, when I wanted to follow up on my immunology work at Yale and study the difference between normal stomach tissue and cancer of the stomach, which was a very common illness at that time. The award was from the National Cancer Institute for $1,000 to help buy laboratory equipment and supplies. (The award letter was signed by Dr. Ralph Meader, who knew me from his days in Dr. Burr's neuroanatomy department at Yale.) I thought I was the world's wealthiest researcher when I got that money. I was able to find a corner of some laboratory where I could work on nights off and on weekends.

Over the course of the next year or two it became apparent that in order to make any progress in a pure science such as tissue immunology I would have to devote my entire lifetime to it; this became especially clear after I visited Dr. Pressman, an immunologist at the Sloan-Kettering Memorial Institute. So I fell back on things I could do and see, areas where I could get publishable results, in addition to pursuing my surgical career. My subsequent grants from the NIH were all in thrombotic vascular disorders. I was fortunate in having numerous surgical residents who wanted to work with me in the laboratory part-time, and we had many varieties of projects going on. We ended up with close to one hundred publications. Among the projects we worked on was coronary artery arteriography, which was published in 1957. Although we had developed a technique for diagnosing occlusive disease of the coronary arteries, there was not much to be done about it at that time because open-heart surgery was not developed until the mid-sixties.

The more widespread prevalence of blood clots in the venous system and the emboli to the lungs led to our learning more about blood clots in the arterial system, particularly when they coexisted throughout the vascular system. One of the puzzles that emerged was the concomitant cause of arterial spasm and gangrene in syndromes dubbed with such mysterious titles as "phlegmasia cerulea dolens." The question of arterial spasm due to blood clot platelet breakdown was raised. Platelets contained serotonin; was it possible that this chemical was the culprit? Our laboratory geared up to measure blood platelet serotonin and its urinary breakdown product 5-hydroxy indol acetic acid (5HIAA) in patients with thrombotic disorders and patients without these disorders. Although nothing definitive was discovered, we became known as the "serotonin laboratory" at Duke.

Coincidentally there emerged a new family of disease—carcinoid tumors, which have an overabundance of serotonin products in them. For years, a benign tumor at the tip of the appendix noted at incidental appendectomy was known to be a carcinoid. It was now discovered that carcinoid tumors could occur in the intestinal tract and subsequently in the bronchial tree with significant potential for malignancy and metastasis. We were fortunate that two patients were referred to us with bronchial carcinoids so that we could study the hormonal aspects of the disease, and that we were able to report our findings in the world literature. Before I knew it, I had became an expert in carcinoid tumors: Dr. David Sabiston, the third chairman of the Department of Surgery at Duke, asked me to write the chapter on carcinoid tumors and serotonin metabolism in several editions of his *Textbook of Surgery*. My experience with research illustrates how one thing can lead to another, by a process of hard work, planning, and being in the right place at the right time. The moral of the story is that one can never appreciate, as a medical student, the importance of a particular research project. Whereas none of my research led to a Nobel Prize, it did open the door for me and many of my next-generation colleagues to savor the challenging field of medical research.

The entire place of research in medical school has changed drastically in the past fifty years. Whereas as a new clinician in the middle of the twentieth century you could have a reasonable and externally fundable and viable research program, it is no longer possible to do so without the equivalent of an M.D.-Ph.D. degree and a commitment to relinquish the practice of clinical medicine or surgery in favor of the laboratory.

I was helped immeasurably during this period by a Markle scholarship. The scholarship was worth $30,000, paid out at the rate of $6,000 a year over five years, to be used in any way the institution wanted to support the work of its Markle scholar. Six thousand dollars was a lot of money in 1953, especially if you had learned to live on $25 a month, as many of us had. In my own case, Dr. Hart put $3,000 toward my salary (which was about $5,000 at that time) and the other $3,000 toward support of my laboratory. It represented a very significant amount of money for me and a major step in my career. I was operating under something of a disadvantage at the time inasmuch as I was still a resident in surgery. (You were supposed to

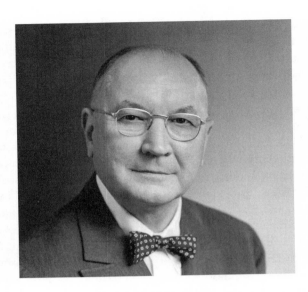

6 Mr. John Russell, president of the Markle Foundation of New York, one of Dr. W. G. Anlyan's mentors in the world of academic medicine. From personal archive of author.

have finished your residency training to be eligible for a Markle scholarship, but somehow I had slipped under the wire because the residency took six years.) Dr. Hart had had to get me an appointment as an assistant professor so I could be eligible, when the more senior residents only had the title of instructor or associate. It led to some hard feelings with my fellow residents.

The John and Mary Markle Foundation was set up in 1927 by a family that had made its fortune in the coal business in Pennsylvania. In 1946 John Russell, who was not a physician but a professional in the world of philanthropy, became president of the Markle Foundation. He assumed this post just as it became apparent that there would be a great boom in the medical world, both in needs to be met and in our ability to meet these needs with new manpower, new knowledge, new techniques, and new drugs.

John Russell spent the first year or so on his new job going around to universities and medical centers, asking how a small amount of money ("a few million a year") could be used to help further medical education in this country and Canada. He was looking for the best possible multiplier effect for the funds he had available. One of the people Russell consulted was

Gene Stead, the chairman of medicine at Duke, and Dr. Stead persuaded Russell that the best investment he could make would be to support young people who were in transition from their residency training to careers in academic medicine. It would be a program to help train a new generation of leaders in academic medicine.

In 1948 the Markle Foundation invited fifty or sixty medical schools in the country each to nominate a single candidate for consideration for a Markle scholarship. Duke nominated Dr. Ivan Brown as its candidate, and he was subsequently selected for the first class of Markle scholars. In 1953 Duke nominated me.

The selection process was precise. First, each medical school had to decide on its candidate. One or more departments would suggest a nominee, and within the medical school a decision would be made about who would represent it that year. Biographical data on the candidate would be submitted to the foundation by May. The Markle people would then invite about forty out of the seventy or eighty candidates to four regional meetings. The regional meeting I went to was in Williamsburg, Virginia—I had never been in such plush surroundings as the Williamsburg Inn. There were about a dozen of us there, and about four or five were going to get the award in each region.

The three-day meeting consisted of a series of private chats with corporate executives, university officers, and foundation administrators, all people who were used to judging others by interviews. The interviewers were there with their spouses. We had breakfast, lunch, cocktails, and dinner together. John Russell said that the British government used this method to pick its intelligence agents during the Second World War. We candidates also got to know one another in this period, and I was sure that, of the twelve people who spent three days at Williamsburg with me, ten were better than I was.

When we went home we did not know whether we had made the cut or not. John Russell attended each meeting, and he gave a subtle hint of how things had gone. No one was supposed to say anything until after receiving a formal letter from the foundation about a month later. To my surprise and delight, I was among those offered a scholarship.

If you were among the chosen in your region, you were invited to New York for dinner with George Whitney, chairman of the board of the Markle Foundation. You were supposed to tell Mr. Whitney in twenty-five words or less what you did every day, which was quite a chore, since the old man was rather deaf. We were all to arrive at seven o'clock, not one minute earlier, not one minute later. The chairs in the large living room in his apartment where we met were arranged in a semicircle around Mr. Whitney, who sat at the head. One Markle scholar-to-be took off on his subject, which was the study of a particular enzyme in biochemistry, and spoke for five or six minutes. Everybody was squirming, knowing that, even though Mr. Whitney was nodding graciously, he probably had not heard a single word. When this scholar sat down at the end of his presentation, Mr. Whitney said, 'Thank you very much, Doctor. Now tell me, what is an enzyme?" At the end of that session, the group, who came from all over the United States and Canada, were told that they had been appointed Markle scholars.

This was before women were even considered as candidates, and so the luncheon preceding the Whitney dinner was held at the Century Association in New York. It being 1953 they would not let women through the front door, so Dorothy Rowden, John Russell's invaluable assistant, was excluded.

Starting in 1953 the Markle Foundation initiated another part of the program: once a year, all Markle scholars were invited to a national meeting to discuss topics of special interest—not necessarily topics related to medicine, but broad social issues that placed medicine in the wider context of the world it serves. The first such meeting took place at Columbia University's Arden House in Harriman, New York. The discussions were lively: we would stay up until one in the morning arguing with one another, and then get up early the next day to continue. This went on for a three-day period, with some authority in each field leading the discussions. The meeting in Aspen in 1957 coincided with the launching of Sputnik. The entire group was jarred to learn that the Soviets were ahead of us in anything related to science, and it became the dominant subject of the conference. Sputnik also, of course, was the incentive for the enormous surge in U.S. scientific research, and the funding for research, in the following decades.

During the course of that year's meeting, John Russell asked me to examine his wife, Hortense. She had recently had a radical mastectomy and a skin grafting of the chest wall by a surgeon at Columbia-Presbyterian who was a world authority in breast cancer. Hortense's complaint was about dryness of the skin graft, which was not unusual at Aspen's altitude. While examining her as taught by my mentors at Duke, I did a more complete examination of the neck, the axillae, and the supraclavicular areas, as well as the chest wall. To my surprise, she had a large metastatic lymph node on the opposite side of the neck to where her mastectomy had been. She had been checked by her physician at Columbia about three weeks earlier.

I asked her whether anybody had examined her neck, and she said no. The dilemma facing me was what I, a mere assistant professor of surgery, should tell Hortense, when a world-renowned expert in breast surgery had not examined her properly for a follow-up? I explained the problem to her in general terms and suggested strongly that she return to New York and visit her doctor as soon as possible. I explained the situation in more precise detail to John Russell and Dorothy Rowden. The reason for including Dorothy in this more intimate information was that John Russell was prone to alcoholic binges, and I never knew how much he would recall when he was under the influence. I knew if I mentioned it to Dorothy, it would be taken care of. Six months after Aspen, Hortense unfortunately developed a large metastatic lesion of the spine and died shortly thereafter.

These annual Markle scholar meetings were especially important as a way to meet people in fields besides surgery. I had been able to meet older surgeons and younger surgeons before, but here I could meet people in anatomy and pediatrics and all the fields of medicine. This was exceedingly helpful when I became dean, because by then I knew people from all disciplines. I knew them on a first-name basis, and I could call on them for input into our selection of faculty. I realized that these were individuals who could be future deans and department chairmen, a reservoir of talented people who had been sifted out by their own institutions and by national selection.

One other advantage of the Markle experience was that John Russell and Dorothy Rowden became our professional father and mother figures. Anytime we wanted advice, personal or professional—"Look, I am being offered this job, what do you think? To whom should I talk?"—they were very helpful.

While the Markle program was important to institutions like Hopkins and Harvard in strengthening their talent pool, it was of even greater importance to younger institutions such as Duke that had not yet built up an endowment. The Markle program helped Duke retain some of its most promising young faculty: people such as Ivan Brown, our first Markle scholar (who later joined the Watson Clinic in Lakeland, Florida) and pediatrician Bill DeMaria, who was Duke's Markle scholar the year ahead of me and who subsequently joined the Duke faculty.

Duke's later Markle scholars included Dr. Andrew Wallace, a cardiologist who was one of the pioneers in finding a treatment for Wolff-Parkinson-White syndrome, a form of cardiac arrhythmia. Wallace nailed down the alterations of the conduction pathways of the heart. Working in collaboration with surgeon Bill Sealy, they developed a technique to interrupt the bad fibers that could cause fibrillation. Andy also initiated Duke's highly successful DUPAC (Duke University Preventive Approach to Cardiology) program, a supervised exercise and lifestyle regimen that has helped thousands of patients through the years. Wallace went on to become director of Duke University Hospital and then dean and head of the Hitchcock Medical Center at Dartmouth. There was considerable prestige attached to being selected chairman of the planning committee for the annual meeting of the scholars, choosing the guest speakers and organizing the meeting. Andy Wallace chaired the final annual meeting of the Markle scholars, and everyone who had ever been part of it was invited back. The program was disbanded shortly after that. In 1999 all living Markle scholars and their spouses were invited for a reunion celebration in Scottsdale, Arizona. It was wonderful to see the survivors and friends of long standing. Each had made a mark in academic medicine.

A study has been done of those who were nominated but not chosen for a Markle scholarship, and, although I did not see the report, I understand that the unsuccessful candidates did not fare much better or much worse than the successful candidates and that by and large they had successful careers as well. But they missed the wonderful fellowship with some very stimulating contemporaries. I think some of them always felt defensive or resentful because they were not chosen, and perhaps they felt that they had let their institutions down, all of which is regrettable.

When John Russell retired as head of the Markle Foundation in the early sixties, Lloyd Morrisett, who had been with the Carnegie Foundation, succeeded him, and the trustees gave him the power to select a field of concentration. He was not particularly enamored of the Markle Scholars Program, and although several of us tried to persuade him that it had had a tremendously beneficial effect on American medical education, he discontinued it after the last five-year class's obligations had been met and decided to focus the foundation's efforts on communications. I have learned that the incoming president of a foundation may change the entire programmatic direction of the philanthropy with the support of its board. A trust, such as The Duke Endowment, is different: it must maintain the original scope of the donor, within reasonable limits.

I felt that the disbandment of the Markle Scholars Program was a terrible loss to the medical world, and in the seventies, when the Searle Family Foundation asked for programmatic direction, I persuaded them to reinstitute a program like that of the Markle scholars. By that time the price tag had gone up from $6,000 a year to something like $35,000 to $40,000, and the focus was mainly on the basic sciences, not on the broad picture of medicine in society that the Markle program gave its participants. The Searle Scholars have an annual meeting, as did the Markle program, where there is a healthy exchange of views and information. When the Lucille P. Markey Charitable Trust came along with monies that had to be expended, they were so impressed with the Searle Scholars Program that they instituted the Markey Scholars Program at $100,000 a year (a lot of it going for equipment and support). After that, the Pfizer Company Foundation came along and said, if Searle had a scholars program, Pfizer had to have one, too. The Pfizer program is financed by the pharmaceutical company, while the Searle program is funded by the family. These other foundations or corporations have together, in different ways, continued the work that was started by the Markle Foundation.

When somebody today asks who our potential deans of medical schools are, we cannot fall back on a reservoir of bright people, in a variety of disciplines, that was fostered by the Markle program. When I became a dean and a member of the Association of American Medical Colleges (AAMC), I knew all the other deans who had been Markle scholars. They also knew Duke and its people. There was a sort of collegial bond; you had a common background from which you could work.

The Markle Scholars Program played a vital role in my own career. Not only did it provide an invaluable network of professional contacts and the opportunity for exchange of ideas but the grant money itself enabled me to stay on at Duke. If I had not received the Markle money in 1953, I could not have supported my research when I finished my residency. I had some NIH grants, but the support coming to me from the Markle Foundation via the university was substantial and justified my staying on. I was not just another resident about whom the question would inevitably be asked, Should we keep him or ship him out? It was not so obvious that I would have been retained, had I not been a Markle scholar. I had gained some notoriety as the person who had recommended the reorganization of the emergency room and the recruitment of interns and house staff. Any time you become known for making decisions that require people to give up power and prestige and to change their way of doing things, you are likely to incur their wrath, and they will work to remove you. But the Markle scholarship protected me, for, in 1955, at the conclusion of my residency, Dr. Hart appointed me, along with Ivan Brown, to five-eighths-time positions at the Veterans Administration Hospital across the road—an appointment that expired when my scholarship did, in 1958.

I passed the general surgical boards in 1955 and the thoracic boards in 1956. In 1958 my three-year appointment at the VA ended, as did my Markle scholarship. In anticipation of the possibility that I be asked to leave, I had visited San Francisco to explore two prospects: first, Vic Richards, then chief of surgery at Stanford, wanted me to look over the chief of surgery job at the VA in San Francisco, and secondly, my older brother—who is also board-certified in general and thoracic surgery, but whose specialties are in cancer—had invited me to join him in private practice. I made a quick visit to the West Coast, but neither offer really appealed to me. I had by then acquired a number of NIH grants and built up a private practice within the PDC, a combination that probably made it possible for Dr. Hart to keep me on. I don't believe we ever had a formal discussion; things just continued, and, since I was not specifically told to leave, I just kept quiet and stayed on.

4

FIRST YEARS AS SURGEON
AND ADMINISTRATOR

B Y   T H E   T I M E I was practicing medicine and beginning my years as a hospital administrator, tremendous changes were taking place in research and the development of new drugs and procedures, as well as in the delivery and practice of medicine, and Duke was in the midst of it all, instigating, implementing, and furthering those changes. There was a surge in research, particularly in trauma, as a result of World War II. Faster transportation, particularly air transportation, meant we could also get wounded, injured, and critically ill patients to hospitals faster. Great advances had been made in blood banking and transfusions. The discovery of sulfanilamide shortly before the war, and of penicillin in 1940–41, gave us the ability to fight infections as never before. With the age of antibiotics coming soon after the discovery of penicillin, and the treatment of tuber-culosis with streptomycin and subsequently with isoniazid, it appeared as though infectious diseases were on their way out.

Apart from the advances in medicine came the growth in third-party in-surance, which had been introduced in the early thirties. It made access to medical care possible for many people to whom it would have been an un-attainable luxury before. The tireless head of the Duke hospital and Medi-cal School, Dr. Wilburt Davison, had been instrumental in the evolution of North Carolina Blue Cross-Blue Shield in the 1930s. At first the Ameri-can Medical Association considered it a socialist move and condemned it. However, it proved to be a major step in the right direction. Also as a result of World War II, officials of the Veterans Administration took a new look at their medical and health care system and determined that they should build all-new VA hospitals as close to university hospitals and academic medical centers as possible, not out in the hinterlands just to please some powerful politicians. Thus the VA hospitals could share the medical centers' clinical faculty and staff and be used for teaching medical students, thereby providing a major expansion for academic programs. Dr. Davison was closely involved in these deliberations. That law was passed in 1948, and late in 1949, the year I got to Duke, they broke ground for the VA Hospital, across the street from the future North Division of Duke University Hospital.

At about that same time, the Hill-Burton Act came along. Good rural hospitals were rare then, and those that existed were falling apart. Senator Lister Hill and Representative Claude Burton were key leaders in remedying that lack.

Following World War II we saw the exponential growth of the National Institutes of Health. The NIH began with some left-over money from a program for venereal disease when the unspent money, instead of being turned back to the federal government, was used for research in nonvenereal disease. With the advent of Dr. James Shannon as director of the NIH, and with the efforts of Senator Hill and Representative John Fogarty, the NIH budget grew substantially, funding research at Duke Medical Center, among other institutions nationwide. The evolution of the NIH was undoubtedly supported by Duke's Dr. Davison. However, his principal contribution in that part of the medical/governmental world was as a member of the Board of Regents of the National Library of Medicine, which had evolved from the old Army Medical Library. (Dr. Barnes Woodhall, head of neurosurgery and later vice provost, was also a regent of the NLM in his time and subsequently chairman of its board of trustees; in the early 1970s, I followed Davison's and Woodhall's footsteps.)

The fifties were also a period of great institutional change at Duke's medical school and hospital. The first generation of chairmen started to phase out, and a new generation came in. Educational and research programs grew, as did the numbers of students and faculty. There was physical growth, but it was haphazard, with a bump here and a bump there, enclosing a courtyard here and a courtyard there. Soon, there would be greater and more logically channeled growth.

At the university level there was conflict, and it centered on the planned evolution of the university. The main protagonists were Hollis Edens, president of Duke University, and Paul M. Gross, the nationally renowned chemist, who had been one of the guiding forces in atomic research at Oak Ridge and who was then dean of the university and vice president for educational affairs. The dispute between them was about whether Duke should continue as a relatively small university focused on undergraduate education (the Edens position) or grow into a major research university competing with Stanford and Yale (Gross's point of view). At the time, there was talk of Dr. Davison becoming president of the university, but it was feared that he was too much in the Gross camp. Both Edens and Gross eventually resigned under pressure from the trustees, and in 1960 Dr. Deryl Hart became acting president of Duke University as a compromise candidate. While all this was roiling the university, the Medical School and hospital were also changing.

Wilburt Davison retired in 1960. He had started at Duke in 1927, and essentially his role was that of dean of a four-year medical school. The dean's office had nothing to do with regulating and overseeing the internship and residency training programs; Davison had left that to the departmental chairmen, wearing their hats as chiefs of service—which is pretty much what his counterparts across the nation also did.

Davison did not go through committees or a bureaucracy; his was an authoritarian style. For example, I had as my patients a husband and wife, very famous people in North Carolina, both of whom needed to come into the hospital. The hospital administrator insisted that husband and wife have separate rooms because the sexes could not be mixed in a semiprivate room. The husband said, "I have been sharing a bedroom with my wife for over fifty years; why can't we be together? We can support each other." As their physician, I said, "Well, it sounds good to me," but the administrator kept saying no. So I called Dr. Davison on the phone; he called the administrator; and we had a new rule: a husband and wife could share the same semiprivate room.

Davison functioned on a very small budget. In the early years, he had been chairman of pediatrics as well as dean, and in my experience, when a dean concomitantly holds a chair in a department, that department will become either very rich or very poor. In Davison's case, he starved pediatrics. They had no full-time or geographic full-time practitioners, and there was no attempt to build a large department. Instead, Davison depended on just three doctors, Jay Arena, Angus McBryde, and Arthur London, all of them private practitioners in Durham who had courtesy clinical appointments; all private patients were referred to them. Later, Davison appointed to his faculty Dr. Jerry Harris (in the latter years, Jerry essentially ran the department) and Dr. Bill DeMaria. With DeMaria's appointment, the door was opened to the gradual recruitment of younger faculty.

Davison also ran the dean's office with minimal funding. Just to throw the annual graduation party for the seniors, he would go each year, hat in hand, to the PDCs to pay for a barbecue at Turnage's, a well-loved but not very expensive Durham institution. That was something I did not want to do when I became dean; it was one of the major reasons why I helped found the Davison Club, the Medical Center's $1,000-a-year support group, and a few other groups to help fund the Medical Center's affairs in an appropriate fashion. The dean's office desperately needed some liquid assets.

In his last years as dean, Davison became more interested in developing primary care services in North Carolina. He became disenchanted with Phil Handler, chairman of biochemistry, and with Gene Stead, chairman of medicine, because he had the feeling that the two of them were leading the Medical School and hospital in the direction of a tertiary-care, research-oriented institution, rather than paying attention to the general or family practitioner. Incidentally, I think he was right that we had not paid enough attention to family practice, and we paid the price for that in the 1960s. (This was one of the reasons I supported the formation of a new Department of Community Health Science in 1966, which subsequently became the Department of Community Medicine and Family Practice in 1972. It met with a lot of resistance on the part of the established strong specialties such as medicine and surgery, which feared that the new department would cut into their patient base. Interestingly, Dr. Stead in his later years dropped his opposition to primary care and became a champion.)

Since Dr. Davison tended to be rather autocratic, some of the department chairmen had suggested that there be a more formal administrative structure. When I got to Duke in 1949, an executive committee was therefore in place, consisting mainly of department chairmen. Dr. Davison subsequently expanded the composition of the executive committee to include the dean of nursing, the superintendent of the hospital, some faculty members, and others who would be invited occasionally to a meeting; it was then called the Committee on Health Affairs. But Dr. Davison was away a great deal in the fifties, and the institution ran essentially on autopilot, with major guidance from Drs. Stead, Hart, and Handler.

In 1959 a search committee was established to find a successor for Dr. Davison. Phil Handler, chairman of biochemistry, was on the committee, as was Barnes Woodhall, chairman of neurosurgery. The group

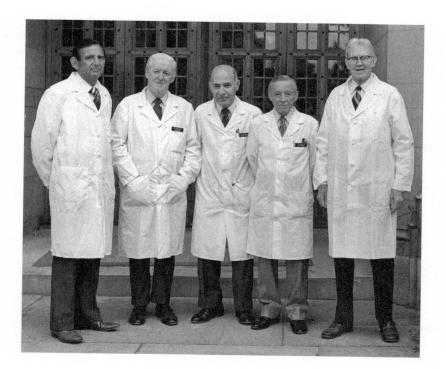

7 A rare moment in Duke's history: some of its early leaders in front of the Davison Building on the university's main campus. (L–R): Dr. Ewald W. Busse, then dean of the Medical School and former chairman of psychiatry; Dr. Thomas D. Kinney, immediate past dean of the school and former chairman of pathology; Dr. W. G. Anlyan; Dr. Barnes Woodhall, second dean of the school, former chancellor of the university and professor of neurosurgery; and Dr. Deryl Hart, president emeritus of Duke University and former chairman of the Department of Surgery. 1974. DUMC Photography.

brought some remarkably weak candidates, one of whom I had known from his days at Yale. Eventually the search committee came to their collective wits and decided they hadn't seen anybody as good as one person on the committee, so they offered the deanship to Barnes Woodhall. He accepted.

Dr. Woodhall was a man of great intelligence and of tremendous integrity. He called a spade a spade, he did not tolerate fools, and he didn't horse around with politics. He was a very heavy cigarette smoker, but he never had the decency to have a cigarette cough (and he did not die of lung cancer but of a debilitating brain disease). The very first thing he did every morning when he came in at five minutes to eight was to get a Coca-Cola and smoke another cigarette in his office. It was a ritual.

Barnes Woodhall's strong suits were neurosurgery and academic work. He was not particularly suited for administrative work. He had an amazing gift, however; he would say something in a meeting, especially to lay people from the outside, and everybody loved what he said, but if you asked them, "What did he really say?" they couldn't tell you. There was another little trick I learned from him. If he was going into a meeting that he knew would be tedious, he would arrange to be paged. Everyone assumed that it was because he had a sick patient. I also learned from Dr. Woodhall that it was important to keep your hand in clinical practice. After all, if you didn't succeed as an administrator, you had a position to go back to. It also kept you current with clinical medicine and made you move through the clinics and wards so that you were approachable by any member of the staff.

It was Dr. Woodhall's dream to develop the north end of the medical campus in a more orderly fashion that led to the studies of how to do it. He persuaded the university trustees of the importance of these plans. As I have told many people, Dr. Woodhall was a dreamer, and I fulfilled his dreams.

Dr. Hart, in his long-standing relationship with me, was very generous. In 1961, when he and Taylor Cole, the first provost of the university, with the concurrence of vice provost Frank de Vyver, felt they needed some fresh blood to head up the university planning committee, they called on me to chair the group. At the time I was just being made a full professor of surgery. This was also about the time of the Berlin crisis and the Cuban missile crisis, and Taylor Cole asked me to head up a "fall-out preparedness committee" for the university. The committee was formed in anticipation of a possible atomic or hydrogen bomb attack on Oak Ridge, which, given the prevailing winds, could have sent a high fall-out of radioactivity to the Durham area. I assume that in large measure my appointment to that committee had come about because I had been the Medical Education for National Defense (MEND) coordinator for the Medical School.

With that mandate, the committee surveyed all the university buildings on campus to ascertain which ones could serve as fall-out shelters; we had those buildings stocked with enough water and dried food for up to three weeks of inhabitation by Duke faculty, students, and families in the surrounding area. One weekend we had a disaster drill in which fall-out sup-

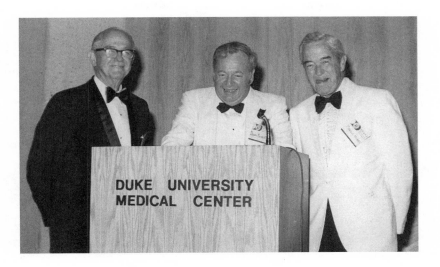

8   On occasion of the Fiftieth Anniversary Emeriti Faculty Dinner, June 10, 1980, three major intrauniversity supporters were welcomed as emeriti faculty of the School of Medicine: (L–R) Dr. R. Taylor Cole, first provost of Duke University (1960) and professor of political science; President Douglas M. Knight, president of Duke 1963–69; and Dr. Marcus Hobbs, former provost and professor of chemistry. DUMC Photography.

posedly was headed our way, and we had to sequester several tens of faculty and students in fall-out shelter simulation. It was my luck to have Taylor Cole, the provost of the university, as one of the people in my shelter, and halfway through the four-hour stretch in the shelter, he became psychotic. We subsequently learned that he was acting on cue with the people who had organized the rehearsal. But we did not know this at the time, so our dilemma was how to deal with this honorable gentleman of high rank who was acting very peculiarly.

By 1963 the Medical Center had grown to such an extent that Duke president Douglas Knight, Provost Taylor Cole, and the trustees felt that there might be room for two people at the head of the Medical Center—one at the vice-presidential level who would relate to the university, and the other, the dean, to concentrate on the internal affairs of the medical center. Following the success of the fall-out preparedness program, Dr. Hart, Provost Cole and Dr. deVyver evidently felt that I might have the potential to assist Dr. Woodhall in running the Medical School. In 1963 Deryl Hart, President

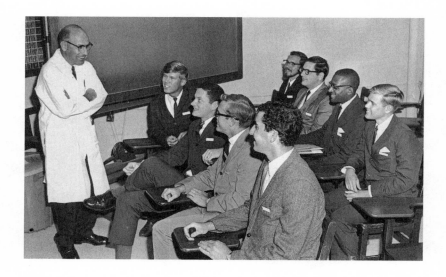

9   Dr. W. G. Anlyan as the new dean, welcoming his first
class of medical students, 1964. DUMC Photography.

Knight, and Provost Cole, with Dr. Woodhall's concurrence, asked me if I
would like to be groomed to become the dean of the Medical School. I felt
rather uneasy, because as an intern and junior resident I had regarded many
of the people making that appointment—Phil Handler and Gene Stead in
particular—as being true international giants, and here I was on the road
to becoming the person they reported to. I was just thirty-eight years old.
The committee made me an associate dean, but unfortunately they forgot
to activate a search committee of chairmen to decide whether I should be
the dean, which created a difficult situation. Another committee was, however, soon established, with Tom Kinney as chairman and Gene Stead, Phil
Handler, and Dan Tosteson as members, and I was formally offered the
deanship in 1964.

When Dr. Woodhall had become dean in 1960, he apparently did not
have a formal governance structure. When I came into the picture as associate dean in 1963, one of the first things some of the department chairmen told me was that we needed a formal structure, and therefore I created
(even before I was appointed dean) a Medical School Advisory Committee
(MedSAC) consisting of all the department chairmen. They did not want
to include the dean of the School of Nursing. I did insist that the director

of the hospital, Charlie Frenzel, be included, so that he would be informed of the MedsAC decisions. I also insisted that the word "advisory" be in the committee's title, because I did not want to be bound by their resolutions. It would have been foolish to set up the committee on any other basis, unless we agreed most of the time. As it turned out, if members did their homework and had talked with key chairmen before the MedsAC meetings, there usually was no major policy disagreement by the time a matter came up for action.

When Dr. Woodhall retired as vice provost in 1969, the Board of Visitors felt that the title "dean of the Medical School" was no longer descriptive of the chief administrator, whose responsibilities had grown well beyond the task of overseeing the four-year Medical School. With the coming of Medicare and Medicaid, that person had also to be on top of the problems of residency training and internship. The hospital was not something to be treated at arm's length by the Medical School but was intrinsic to graduate training, meaning that the Medical School administrator had to be above whoever was running the hospital. There were also the research budgets: the complexities of overseeing all that had grown as well. So it was decided, in 1969, that the title should be changed to "vice president for health affairs"—the title was linked to that of the president of university, so that the university president had a vice president who took care of both the academic Medical Center and of health affairs.

When I became vice president for health affairs in 1969, the question was raised whether I should retain the position of dean of the Medical School. By that time, I had enjoyed on the national scene all the benefits of being dean. As a member of the Association of American Colleges, I had been in a leadership position. I was the first chairman of the Council of Deans when it was formed in Washington in 1968. The title (and position) of dean was not, however, something I particularly wanted to hold onto. Instead, I decided to transfer the deanship responsibilities to someone else and to try an innovation: to change the title of the position to "director of medical education." I picked Thomas Kinney for the position, because he was very highly regarded both by the faculty as well as nationally. Dr. Kinney was kind enough to accept the post, while retaining the chairmanship of the Department of Pathology.

When Tom Kinney retired from his administrative posts at the age of sixty-five—which was mandatory at that time—Dr. Ewald (Bud) Busse took over his responsibilities. Dr. Busse had been chairman of psychiatry for more than twenty years and wanted to give up that position, and I

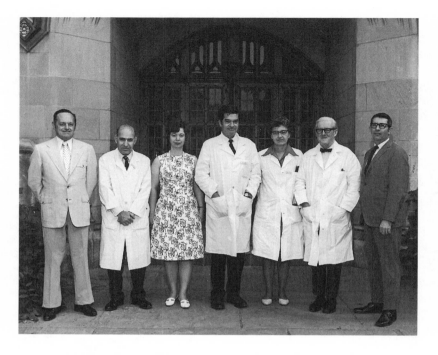

10   The Vice President's Advisory Committee (L–R): Jeff Steinert, assistant vice
president for business and finance; Dr. W. G. Anlyan; Ruby Wilson, dean, School
of Nursing; Stuart Sessoms, director, Duke Hospital; Dr. Jane Elchlepp, assistant
vice president for planning; Dr. Thomas Kinney, director of medical education and
professor of pathology; and James (Pete) Bennett, assistant to the vice president,
May 1972. DUMC Photography.

thought he was a natural to become director. But since Dr. Kinney had
had a difficult time explaining to people on the national scene what a "director of medical education" did, we changed the title to "dean of medical
education." Like Kinney, Busse had responsibility for the Medical School,
from admission to graduation; allied health education; and graduate medical education, although he and the CEO of the hospital worked together on
the internship-residency phase.

   As vice president for health affairs, I appointed, in 1969, a Vice President's Advisory Committee (VPAC), in addition to MedSAC. VPAC included
the dean of the School of Nursing and the director of the hospital, as well as
the top staff, the people in charge of finance and management. Jeff Steinert

was an early member when he was assistant vice president of finance, and after that John Shytle and Bob Winfree served on the committee. Barney McGinty, the medical center controller, and the top staff would also sit in, as would R. C. (Bucky) Waters, representing alumni and development. Waters had been Duke's basketball coach and became a first-rate fund-raiser for the Medical Center. At all of these meetings, every member had the privilege of bringing in whatever agenda item he or she wanted to discuss. If there was anything controversial, they generally talked to me ahead of time.

MedSAC dealt principally with the academic affairs of the Medical School, education and research, whereas VPAC concerned itself across the board with the Medical Center. When I became chancellor for health affairs in 1983, VPAC became the Chancellor's Advisory Committee, or CAC. When I delegated the leadership of the Medical School to Tom Kinney, the director of medical education and subsequently the dean of nursing also became members. There was some overlap between the two committees, but the membership was different. I would never want to put up a huge new building without running it by the Medical Center Advisory Committee, but all the groundwork and preparation for MedSAC and subsequent presentation to the university and the trustees was done by the staff and the CAC meeting.

All appointments and promotions had to go through MedSAC, and I remember some tough discussions about people, usually faculty who had not published very much but who had been on the faculty for a long time and, by their service, deserved promotion. It is interesting that people who were for promotion in some instances were against promotion for people with equal credentials in other instances. Faculty in Harvey Estes's Department of Community and Family Medicine were constantly badgered about their lack of publications. On occasion, some of the other clinical departments had the same problem—longtime clinical faculty who were difficult to promote. In the basic sciences, there was no question some faculty were not worthy of promotion unless they had a good publication record and a good history of NIH or National Science Foundation support. But in the clinical field there are two distinct classes of faculty. The clinical investigators spend much of their time doing research and some teaching, with responsibility for a minimum of clinical care; those faculty—just like the basic scientists—had no problem publishing and being promoted. The tough ones were individuals such as Bill Floyd, as an example, who were the workhorses of cardiology and other fields, who took care of patients fifteen or more hours a day and were at the mercy of telephone calls from their patients. These people just did not have time to publish sufficiently to compare with the clinical investigators. There was no question that it took longer for the pure clinician to be promoted.

I was fortunate during this period to have the friendship and guidance of John Russell, president of the Markle Foundation, whom I met through my association as a Markle scholar. Early in my administrative career, when the Duke University Medical Center's Board of Visitors was being formed under the aegis of Barnes Woodhall, I suggested John Russell as a member. John was a quiet person on the board, but he would always take me aside after the meetings and give me some sound advice. On one occasion he told me exactly how to use the Board of Visitors. He recommended that we mix four or five key university trustees along with people who were experts in the health field, so we could educate the trustees in what we wanted to do. This way, when decisions had to be made, there would be university trustees who would have the background to champion the causes of the Medical Center. This happened very successfully. As a matter of fact, some members of the Board of Visitors who were not trustees to begin with ended up being recommended by me to become members of the Duke University Board of Trustees—people such as Ray Nasher, a very successful land developer in Texas; Karl Bays, the CEO of American Hospital Supply Corporation in Chicago; and Ed Benenson, a real-estate investor from New York. (To this day, some twenty-five years later, Ed Benenson hosts a major luncheon annually for my successor, Dr. Ralph Snyderman, in Palm Beach, thus keeping the important Duke-Florida connection fresh.)

The purpose of the Board of Visitors, as I put it together and nurtured it, was to support the major decisions that lay ahead of the Medical Center. I am told that today an individual has to contribute a large amount of money to qualify for the board, so that it has become part of the development effort, in contrast to giving advice and support for major policy decisions.

One other piece of advice John Russell gave me was to "delegate, delegate, delegate." He believed that the best administrators are the laziest ones, who give everybody else their jobs to do. In my career, whenever I could lump several responsibilities together and hand them to somebody else, I delegated. My personal philosophy was that my time should be spent worrying about tomorrow, not running the institution today. I would concentrate on planning for the future and leave the day-to-day administration of research and clinical practice to the department chairmen, intervening only occasionally, when the decisions entailed policy matters.

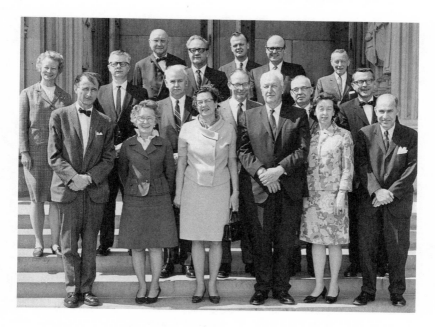

11   The first Duke Medical Center Board of Visitors, 1968. (Front row, L–R): Dr. John N. Pappenheimer, Dr. Ruth Freeman, Miss Florence Julian, Mr. Marshall L. Pickens, Dr. Rozella Schotfeldt, Dr. W. G. Anlyan; (middle row, L–R): Dr. Irene Brown, Dr. Jacob Kooman, Dr. Francis James Braceland, Dr. John B. Hickham, Dr. Ben N. Miller, Dr. Kenneth R. Crispell; (back row, L–R): Mr. John M. Russell, Mr. Richard J. Stull, Dr. John H. Knowles, Dr. Martin M. Cummings, Dr. Barnes Woodhall. DUMC Photography.

I was determined to improve the national ranking of the Duke hospital and Medical School and make it one of the top institutions in the country. It all started in the winter of 1949 during my senior year in medical school at Yale. When I accepted the internship offer in surgery at Duke, some of my classmates asked where it was located. At the time, I was slightly annoyed that they did not immediately recognize it as a high-quality institution. In retrospect, I realize that the Medical School and the hospital had only been in existence for nineteen years and had not had much time to develop a national reputation.

During my residency years, I had the privilege of going to a few national surgical meetings to present research papers—meetings such as the Surgical Forum of the American College of Surgeons, the Society of University Surgeons, and eventually the American Surgical Association. Whereas older, established surgical programs usually had multiple paper presentations, a Duke paper was a relative rarity. At the same time those older schools had many nationally renowned faculty members participating in the meetings. Duke had Dr. Deryl Hart, Dr. Clarence E. Gardner, and the maverick Dr. Keith Grimson in general and thoracic surgery; Dr. Barnes Woodhall in surgical specialties; and Dr. Guy Odom in neurosurgery (our division of neurosurgery was probably one of the best in the country, if not the world, on a par with the Neurologic Institute at McGill in Montreal or with Johns Hopkins). Some other surgical specialties, such as plastic surgery under Dr. Ken Pickrell, were just being recognized on the national scene. But other components of the school and hospital varied in name recognition in the period 1949–50.

The most renowned was Dr. Eugene Stead, who had become chairman of the Department of Medicine in 1946. He had brought with him from Emory several young clinical investigators who became members of the Society for Clinical Investigation and eventually the Association of American Physicians: Frank Engel in metabolism and endocrinology, Jack Myers (subsequently chairman at the University of Pittsburgh), and John Hickam (subsequently chairman at Indiana). Dr. Nick Carter was distinguished in obstetrics-gynecology circles.

In the clinical area, Ewald W. Busse had come from the University of Colorado in Denver in 1953 to become chairman of psychiatry at Duke. Already noted nationally for his interest in neurologic diseases and mental health and aging, he became an outstanding faculty member who commanded everyone's respect. Busse was awarded one of the earliest NIH grants, in 1955, to support the development of the Center for Aging, which has thrived ever since.

However, the two biggest names and programs at Duke were Dr. Walter Kempner, with his rice diet, and J. B. Rhine, with his studies in extrasensory perception (ESP). It was painful to me personally to be quizzed about the latter, since I did not believe in ESP. Dr. Kempner had a legitimate place in my book, since his rice diet was one of the leading treatments at the time for hypertension. Over the years, however, as antihypertensive medications evolved, Kempner used the same rice diet to treat very obese patients, and I did not consider such a program the crown of a highly prestigious institution.

The basic science departments in the late 1940s and 1950s were as much in need of strengthening as the weaker surgical and medical departments. Whereas microbiology had been fortunate to have the individual leadership of Dr. David T. Smith and Dr. Norman Conant, the department needed revitalizing. The same was true of anatomy, where Dr. Joseph Markee had been an innovator in his field but had focused much of his energy on his role of dean of admissions for the Medical School. Pathology's George Margolis, who had been a distinguished neuropathologist under Wiley Forbus's chairmanship, had left some time before to assume the chair at Dartmouth. In microbiology, Norman Conant was highly touted as a mycologist, along with David T. Smith, who had edited *Zinsser's Textbook of Microbiology* for many editions. But they were outstanding individuals rather than an outstanding department.

The exception among the basic sciences was biochemistry, where the chairman, Dr. Philip Handler, had evolved into a major national and international figure and was building up an excellent department. In 1956 Handler and Gene Stead had recruited James Wyngaarden to the Department of Medicine from Washington University in Saint Louis, and in 1957, they asked him to head up the Research Training Program (RTP), which was the predecessor of Duke's M.D.-Ph.D. program.

In addition to being asked, back in the late 1940s, where Duke was located, it was equally frustrating to correct people who thought the name was Drake or something similar. In any event, the late fifties was a time to build our reputation, and build it we did. In general surgery, Dr. Bill Shingleton, who had joined the faculty in the early 1950s, was successful in securing research grants and publishing papers after they were presented at national meetings. At Bill's invitation I had the privilege of collaborating with him on some of his projects and he reciprocated by collaborating on some of mine. Between 1951 and 1956 we were coauthors of twelve published papers. By 1953 I had my own laboratory, and one of my highest priorities was to engage as many of the surgical residents to join me in one or more experimental studies.

The year 1956 was a particularly interesting one. I was then a younger member of the surgical faculty (my appointment had been confirmed in 1955), and with Dr. Hart's support and sponsorship I gave my first paper at the American Surgical Association; it was not an earth-shattering presentation, but it provided me the opportunity for exposure to the most renowned academic surgeons of the United States and Canada, as well as a sprinkling of the notables from abroad. Just one year before, that same meeting introduced the first papers on open-heart surgery done under direct vision with hypothermia. I was utterly fascinated, as a senior resident, hearing history in the making.

It was in 1956 that Dr. Hart, recovering from a mild heart attack, chose to give up operative surgery. He delegated some additional responsibilities to me including the process of recruitment of interns and residents in general surgery. My former co-resident in general and thoracic surgery, Dr. Ivan W. Brown, had also joined the faculty. The two of us had been assigned for five-eighths of our time as assistant chiefs of surgery at the VA Hospital across Erwin Road. These appointments provided us with clinical surgical patients, since in the Duke private system we were still unknown and would have lacked referrals from both within the institution and outside it.

I was deeply impressed that some of the most senior physicians at Duke, people who had access to the senior surgeons, began to refer patients to me. Dr. Stead, Dr. Carter, and many of their colleagues were among those who made such referrals. Later, I would follow their example and request consultations from the youngest and newest faculty in other specialties.

In 1958, at the end of my five-year Markle Scholarship, I was appointed associate professor of surgery. I made it a point to have each resident be the senior author of a publication resulting from the studies we were conducting and to present the paper at the respective surgical meeting. By 1958 we had five papers presented at the Surgical Forum of the American College of Surgeons. Duke was going to be on the map. To add to the momentum, Dr. W. Glenn Young (just finishing his Duke residency) and Dr. Ivan Brown joined Dr. Will Sealy in thoracic surgery. As a team they would develop the Duke open-heart surgery program with excellent national visibility.

The year 1959 was an up-and-down year. It was up because on the home and national front Duke's recognition in academia continued to grow. It was, though, also a slightly down year, because I was invited to lecture in London and Paris and to attend the International Surgical Society meeting in Munich—and in all three places I was, once again, faced with having to explain where Duke University was. However, an offset was that Barnes Woodhall was also in attendance at the Munich meeting, accompanied by his wife, Frances, and their daughter, Betsy, who had been a nursing student at Duke. The meeting gave us the opportunity to meet often, both professionally and socially, and in the course of it we became close colleagues and life-long friends. Barnes generously introduced me to his renowned colleagues, most of whom were neurosurgeons.

In 1960 Dr. Hart became acting president of Duke and turned over the

Department of Surgery to his longtime colleague Dr. Clarence E. Gardner Jr., who had been Dr. Hart's first resident in 1930. As acting chairman Dr. Gardner asked me if I would devote more time to assisting him with the administrative matters of the department.

In 1961 Dr. Gardner promoted me to a full professorship. Appointed along with me was the late Dr. Nicholas Georgiade, my lifelong friend and colleague, a fellow intern in 1950 who was to advance eventually to become chief of plastic and maxillofacial surgery at Duke.

Dr. Woodhall had been named dean of the School of Medicine the previous year, succeeding our founding dean, Dr. Wilburt C. Davison, who retired and became a trustee of The Duke Endowment. The stage was set for Duke as a university to begin to reach for national prominence. President Hart, in his wisdom, picked two people from among the very renowned Duke faculty in the arts and sciences to steer Duke from a regional college to a national and international institution, selecting Dr. Taylor Cole as his provost and Dr. Frank deVyver as his vice provost.

Dr. Cole, a noted scholar of German who had obtained his Ph.D. from Harvard in the thirties, was a political scientist of international stature. (I used to kid him about his Texas roots.) Though he would never admit it, he was reported to have been our "chief spy" stationed in Stockholm during World War II. He apparently made several sorties into Germany during the war. Needless to say, his boldness and bravery came with him into the newly created office of the provost. A quiet and very soft-spoken man, he was firm in his missions for the university. He introduced the concept of boards of visitors at Duke—a program that had impressed him at Harvard. This opened the door to inviting a whole new cadre of scholars, government officials, foundation heads, and other important personae to visit Duke on a regular basis to provide advice and consultation in a designated area. (The Medical Center under Dr. Woodhall formed its first Board of Visitors in 1963—as a new associate dean, I played a small part in its organization.) The whole program of boards of visitors throughout selected components of the university brought it additional visibility on the national and international scene.

Dr. Frank deVyver was a labor economist. In contrast to Dr. Cole he was an extrovert; everybody loved "Uncle Frank." Both deVyver and Cole were peacemakers and negotiators, each with his own style. I regarded them both as important mentors of mine.

Hart, Cole, and deVyver formed a solid team, and in 1963 they persuaded the trustees of the university that the time had come to end segregation.

What a transformation—African American students were admitted and black faculty were sought. All the wards in Duke Hospital were opened up to patients regardless of race. We got rid of the dual sets of toilets, water fountains, and morgues. No longer would Duke be regarded as inferior to the Ivy League or the other well-known universities in the country.

5

BUILDING THE DUKE MEDICAL
SCHOOL FACULTY

WHEN I BECAME dean in 1964, the Duke University Medical Center was still not one of the top ten academic medical centers in the country. There had been some improvements in the early sixties. Dr. Philip Handler, chairman of biochemistry, had helped recruit Dr. Dan Tosteson as chair of physiology-pharmacology, and together they had helped persuade Dr. Thomas D. Kinney to succeed Dr. Wiley Forbus as chairman of pathology. Kinney arrived from Case Western Reserve, where he had been a key instigator of curricular changes at its medical school, bringing with him such people as Nathan Kaufman and Don Hackel.

But there was still work to be done. Pediatrics had Jerry Harris as chairman, but the department was not particularly distinguished. Obstetrics-gynecology had some stars in a reasonably good department, under the chairmanship of Bayard (Nick) Carter, but there was no fundamental research going on (with the exception of the endocrinology research of Edwin C. Hamblen, who did not often see patients). Dr. Davison used to refer jokingly to ob-gyn as the "mechanical department."

There was justification for not ranking the Medical School, as a corporate whole, among the top ten. Since I am a poor loser and like to be at the head of the class (a trait instilled in me by my parents, who would never accept my being second in any of my courses), I felt that Duke had all the potential to be number 1 but had not quite made it.

However, I was very fortunate to come to the helm of the Medical Center during a golden age of academic medicine. NIH support was plentiful for those who merited it. We were blessed with the signing in 1965 of Medicare and Medicaid, thanks to the leadership of President Lyndon Johnson. This helped people who needed medical care to get it—and expanded our patient base in the process; it also augmented the funds available for medical education. Under President Richard Nixon we got the National Cancer Act, which expanded the funding available for cancer research and cancer care. Duke jumped to the forefront of cancer research under the leadership of Bill Shingleton, Bill Joklik, and Wayne Rundles. Simultaneously, development programs were evolving in all institutions to raise money from private sources, and each academic medical center and university had well-defined development offices.

In 1972, as we prepared to build the North Division of Duke University Hospital, there were no tax-exempt bond issues in North Carolina; when it came to funding the hospital, we had to do it with private bond placement. But we wrote the issues in such a way that they could be converted to tax-exempt bonds when the necessary legislation was passed, and Duke took the lead in developing tax-exempt bonding for both educational institutions and health facilities within the state. I used to commute to New York, because the best bond lawyers for North Carolina were based on Wall Street. They were able to get the law passed by the North Carolina legislature shortly after the opening of the North Division, so we converted the base funding from private placement to tax-exempt bonds. With tax-exempt bonds, funding large projects became much more feasible.

For all of these reasons, in the "golden age" bigger was better, as long as you maintained control over quality. Growth without quality is a self-defeating exercise. So in everything we did, the ultimate goal was to assure that quality remained high, even—or especially—as the institution grew. One level of quality control is to watch the people the chairmen recruit and how they fit into the organization. Just as the chairmen were the best people I could find, they had to hire the best they could find. The chairmen of the individual departments also kept a day-to-day surveillance over quality in education and in patient care. An additional quality control mechanism was the constant feedback from people in other departments dealing with a particular group—as when I had had a lot of complaints about the quality of cardiac surgery at Duke, particularly pediatric surgical care, which led to the recruitment of Dave Sabiston, a highly regarded pediatric cardiac surgeon.

We also depended on external reviews for quality control. The feedback on a site visit and what outside experts felt about the program were very important considerations. Various boards of visitors included lay people who provided feedback on quality as seen from the eyes of the consumer. In the research areas, quality assurance was a by-product of peer review by the NIH and the National Science Foundation (NSF).

As changes were made at the top of the Medical Center administration, a changing of the guard in the chairmanships was also taking place. When I was still an associate dean, in 1963, it was apparent that we were going to have to replace many of the chairmen of the academic departments in the Medical School. I felt that the way to overhaul the quality of the Medical School was to get really outstanding leadership among the chairmen, where most of the field command was exercised.

The most important thing I learned early in the game was to go out and find the very best person for a given job. I always looked for the best in the country or the best in the world, and, unless they made outrageous demands, in most cases we were able to meet their needs in terms of money, space, support, and administrative structure to recruit the people we wanted. I tried to look for people who were thirty-five to thirty-eight years old and had their futures ahead of them. They might be a little bit of a gamble, but they had to have chalked up an excellent track record. I did not want to recruit people who regarded Duke as a nice place to retire.

My basic philosophy in dealing with people is that 85 percent of any individual is good and 15 percent is bad, and you have learn how to deal with the 85 percent. Admittedly, there are some people whose bad 15 percent is right up front, and it is sometimes difficult to get past it, but that did not keep me from trying to find the good 85 percent in the variety of people needed to work together.

To the credit of my predecessors, Dan Tosteson and Tom Kinney were already aboard, and they, along with Phil Handler, were extremely helpful in attracting subsequent basic science chairmen, such as David Robertson in anatomy and Wolfgang Joklik in microbiology.

Roy Parker, in obstetrics-gynecology, was the first chairman I appointed. Nick Carter was going to retire, and Roy Parker had been the executive officer of the department for a number of years and was the logical candidate from the inside. We did not meet any resistance in making that appointment.

The second position I had to fill was the chairmanship in surgery. When Deryl Hart became president of Duke University in 1960, Clarence Gardner was appointed acting interim head of the Department of Surgery; the powers-that-be apparently thought Dr. Hart would return to the department after serving as president, and therefore kept the chairmanship open for him for three years. Dr. Gardner and I had a close father-son relationship, and we worked well together in running the department.

By the winter of 1964 the clamor for finding a new chairman of surgery was pretty loud. Especially wanting was pediatric cardiac surgery: the pediatricians were not pleased with the capabilities of the surgeons in the division of thoracic surgery, and they were beginning to refer their patients elsewhere. Starting in February 1964 I began the process of looking for a chair for surgery. This was not too difficult, since I had grown up with many of the outstanding young people in the field. While Bill Shingleton and I were at the Society of University Surgeons meeting in Los Angeles, we interviewed James Maloney of UCLA and came back and reported to a small ad hoc committee that included Gene Stead. A month later, I went up to Johns Hopkins to take a look at Dave Sabiston; we had grown up together as young men in academic surgery.

It was Duke's good fortune that Dr. Sabiston had not been appointed to succeed his mentor, Alfred Blalock, as chairman of surgery at Hopkins. The Hopkins search committee had instead picked George Zuidema, who was in the Department of Surgery at the University of Michigan. Zuidema offered Dr. Sabiston the position of chief of pediatric surgery at the new children's hospital at Hopkins, but this was not the level of responsibility for which Sabiston had been prepared. (Zuidema, incidentally, did not end up staying long at Hopkins: a few years later, he returned to Michigan as a vice president.)

In the course of a three-day visit to Johns Hopkins I interviewed all of the chairmen who knew Sabiston, including Arnold Rich, the legendary former head of pathology and Sam Asper, professor of surgical pathology. I asked each to address only one point: Sabiston's liabilities. I had grown up with him, and I knew his record. Everyone gave very supportive answers regarding Sabiston's strengths, which far outweighed his liabilities. The only two exceptions were Dr. A. McGhee Harvey, the chairman of medicine, and his former student, the chairman of pathology, Dr. Ivan Bennett. These two chairmen must, I think, have harbored a deep grudge or jealousy against Blalock. They didn't want anyone who looked like Blalock for another twenty to twenty-five years—and Sabiston was clearly a doctor in Blalock's mold. Blalock, however, spent a long time with me in private chats, telling me all the virtues of Dave Sabiston. I know he was very proud of him, and he told me that without question he had hoped that Dave would succeed him as chairman.

When I got back from Baltimore, I invited Dr. Sabiston to come on two visits, one alone and one with his wife, Aggie, to be seen by as many of the other chairmen at Duke as were available. Everyone thought he was wonderful, and so in the spring I invited him to join us as chairman of surgery, and he did so in September 1964. Shortly before, as one of my first acts as dean, I had named Dr. Gardner chairman retroactive to 1960, when he had become acting chairman, so that he would historically be recorded as the second chairman of surgery, and Dr. Sabiston would be the third. In the meantime I asked President Knight if the Sabistons could buy the lot of university-owned land next to mine on Pinecrest Road. Doug Knight agreed, and the Sabistons rented a house nearby for the two years it took to build their new home.

In his nearly thirty years as chair, Dr. Sabiston developed an outstanding Department of Surgery. Many of his residents in general and thoracic surgery ended up as division heads or chairmen of other departments of surgery. In particular, he was extremely fond of Sam Wells, who essentially grew up at Duke and ended up on the faculty. When Dr. Wells was a full professor, he was recruited by Washington University in Saint Louis. I tried to dissuade him from going by offering him the directorship of the Comprehensive Cancer Center, but the position did not have the kind of line authority over budget, space, and training of residents as did a department of surgery, so he went to Saint Louis. Interestingly, Dr. Wells has recently come full circle, moving back to Duke after a short stint at the American College of Surgeons, bringing with him the American College of Surgeons Oncology Group (ACOSOG).

Gene Stead, one of the real giants of Duke University, should be credited with developing a whole generation of clinical investigators. In 1947, when he came from Emory to Duke as chairman of the Department of Medicine, he brought with him some young clinicians who were national investigators in their own rights and who commanded NIH funding for their research programs. They included Jack Myers, who ended up as chairman of the Department of Medicine at Pittsburgh; John Hickam, who became professor of medicine at Indiana; and Frank Engel, who unfortunately died when he was only fifty-one years old in his laboratory in the Bell Building.

Stead is a man who has supported many innovations. For example, in 1965 he came to me to ask if I, as the new dean, would cover his flank if he took on three former medical corpsmen to see how they might fit into the health care system. (He was particularly worried about the reaction of the nurses, who might think he planned to substitute corpsmen for nurses.) He pointed out to me that about 22,000 army medical corps men a year were being discharged from the armed services with nowhere to go in civilian life, unlike airplane pilots, who could readily be employed by the airlines. Shortly after that encounter, I was at a meeting in Arizona of the Board of Regents of the American College of Surgeons, where I encountered one of the navy's surgeon generals. I told him about the 22,000 corpsmen a year being discharged. He didn't believe me, but he came to see me the next day to say that he had checked with the Pentagon and that the figure was indeed correct. That started the physician's assistant program. I remember John Hickam saying one day that Gene Stead is capable in any week of coming up with about ten wild ideas, of which one was worth pursuing, and the challenge was to recognize the one worth pursuing.

Another major figure in reinvigorating the Medical Center at Duke was Dan Tosteson, who joined us in 1961 as the chair of physiology and pharmacology. He came from the Washington University School of Medicine and was closely involved with the NIH. Dan knew quality work, he knew how to write grants, and he got things done. He managed to hold together the combined physiology-pharmacology department, though to some degree at the expense of sustaining a small pharmacology unit and nourishing more generously the physiology component. He was extraordinarily well respected on the national scene.

Dr. Thomas Kinney, the new chair of our Department of Pathology, was very outgoing and effusive—perhaps he had a little bit of the blarney of the Irish—but he was loved by everybody. He was a well-rounded, well-read scholar who was prominent not only in his field of pathology but in all the basic sciences. He wielded considerable power in the Council of the National Institute of General Medical Sciences, and he helped get Duke one of the first grants for an MD.-Ph.D. program.

Jim Wyngaarden, who had been recruited by Handler and Stead in the late fifties, was thoroughly honest, extremely intelligent, unemotional in his business decisions, and set his priorities. When he came to Duke, he was clearly the star in the Department of Medicine; Dr. Stead recognized that and was willing to step out of the chairmanship at the age of fifty-nine to make room for Jim, as Jim was being recruited by other institutions. That transition unfortunately did not take place soon enough, and Wyngaarden went to the University of Pennsylvania, the nation's oldest medical school. But we wanted him back and worked hard to find a way.

At the MedSAC meeting there was ample discussion of the delicacy of the situation. We did not want to be raiding our sister institutions. After all, we had now arrived as a major and exciting institution that was gathering momentum on the path to excellence and national recognition. Since the two most important clinical departments in any school are medicine and surgery, it was important that those two chiefs got along. Medical history is full of examples of conflict between medicine and surgery at nationally prominent medical schools. MedsAC unanimously approved our approach to Jim Wyngaarden; they delegated Dave Sabiston and me to carry out the first step as discreetly as possible, to avoid placing Jim in an embarrassing position in his new post at Penn. Dave and I proposed that the two of us meet Jim in New York in a very private area to assess his degree of interest in returning to Duke.

I arranged the rendezvous at the International Hotel at Kennedy Airport in New York. I would have a private suite. Dave and I would fly to LaGuardia and take a cab to Kennedy. Jim would take the train to New York City and take a cab to the hotel. I had visions of having missed my vocation in the Central Intelligence Agency.

As it turned out, there were numerous acquaintances on the plane between Raleigh-Durham and LaGuardia. Some of them voiced their curiosity as to what Dave and I were up to. The meeting with Jim occurred without further incident. He was definitely interested. To celebrate we took Jim to dinner in the main dining room before returning to our respective bases. The word of our meeting leaked. However, since Jim and his family were thoroughly familiar with Duke and Durham, negotiations did not take long before he agreed to return, just two years after his departure. Also fortuitously, Gene Stead had lived like a Spartan and hoarded his resources, including a substantial endowment. Duke was on a roll, and Jim Wyngaarden became an exemplary leader for his tenure until President Ronald Reagan asked him to become the director of the National Institutes of Health in 1982.

As chairman at Duke, James Wyngaarden was probably the most valuable colleague I had. I always felt the most important chair in any medical school has to be the chair in medicine, because it is so central to the process of medical education at all levels. You could only be as good a school as your Department of Medicine. Jim was first-rate as successor to Gene Stead, who was a phenomenon on his own. Jim was so thoroughly honest that, if he saw something on the agenda of MedsAC that he disagreed with, he would tell me his views privately; I would encourage him to make his views known in executive session. Once a vote was taken, if his point of view was not supported, however, he left the room totally in support

of the institutional position. Jim won national acclaim for bringing attention to the fact that the training of clinical investigators in medicine was
beginning to fall apart and that we needed to address the issue as a nation.

By comparison, filling the chair of obstetrics-gynecology was very
straightforward. When Roy Parker retired from the chairmanship, I wanted
the internal candidate, Chuck Hammond, to get the chair. I had known
him since he was a medical student and an intern in surgery; he was an excellent surgeon, an outstanding specialist, and seemed to be the modern
version of Roy Parker.

The chair of biochemistry in the early years of my deanship was Dr. Phil
Handler. In the fifties he emerged not only as a leader of the faculty in
the basic sciences but also as one of the leaders in the Medical School in
general. When I arrived at Duke in 1949, William (Pearlie) Perlzweig had
been chairman. During my internship year, 1949–50, Dr. Perlzweig came
down with a moderately advanced cancer of the colon, and I was the intern
taking care of him on Dr. Hart's service. The two fair-haired boys in the department were Phil Handler and Hans Neurath. After Dr. Perlzweig died,
Handler was selected to succeed him as chairman. Hans Neurath went to
the new medical school in Seattle. Both Handler and Neurath did well in
the international world of biochemistry; both became prominent on the
Washington scene and members of the National Academy of Sciences.

Phil Handler was very articulate, a brilliant speaker, obviously extremely
intelligent, yet in many ways a humble man, and very respectful. He was
easy to get along with, but you had to deal with him on facts. He had
started out at the City College of New York, had adjusted extremely well to
Duke University, and was a strong champion of the university as a whole.
An intimate friend of Paul Gross, and particularly during the Gross-Edens
debacle in 1959, there was no question where his allegiance lay. Handler
was also a strong Democrat, as was Dan Tosteson. Handler was one of the
campus leaders in the movement to deny Vice President Nixon an honorary degree. He was obviously well respected on the campus. But there
was still an element of sibling rivalry when it came to working with the
Chemistry Department (Gross's bailiwick), which I attributed mostly to
the Chemistry Department's being afraid of having their potential Ph.D.
students wooed away from chemistry to biochemistry. (Incidentally, that
same rivalry seemed to persist when Bob Hill eventually succeeded Phil
Handler.)

During his tenure as chair of biochemistry, Phil Handler became more
and more occupied with Washington and the challenges both at the Na-

tional Institutes of Health, the National Science Foundation, and at the National Academy of Sciences. In the mid-sixties, when the presidency of the National Academy of Sciences was open, he was called to that position, which he held for twelve years. We reserved an office suite in the Nana-line Duke Building for his use after he retired from the NAS, but unfortunately he developed a malignant lymphoma and never made it back to Duke. When Phil left, we chose Bob Hill as chairman of biochemistry.

Wolfgang Joklik was our top candidate for the chairmanship of the Department of Microbiology and Immunology. He is of Austrian descent and had spent his early years in Australia. After World War II he went to Oxford University to get his D.Phil. He was in the cell biology unit at Albert Einstein Hospital when he came to our attention. I recall sitting in a small suite in the Gotham Hotel on 55th Street in New York with Tom Kinney, twisting Joklik's arm to come to Duke. He had already made his first visit to Durham, and ours was a follow-up visit to persuade him to come. At Duke, Joklik did an outstanding job of building microbiology and immunology as a combined department; he also became the successor to D. T. Smith as editor of *Zinsser's Textbook of Microbiology*. Joklik was in the mold in which I recruited people: he was first and foremost a university and medical center citizen, and secondly charged with building the department he headed with the resources that were available. He was also the key chairman to develop the basic science component of our comprehensive cancer center.

David Robertson was associate professor of neuropathology in the Department of Neurology and Psychiatry at Harvard Medical School when we recruited him. He was a breath of fresh air and willing to go along with the new curriculum as it was being developed, which meant trimming the number of teaching hours of gross anatomy from something like four hundred hours during the first year of medical school to less than one hundred. This was heresy to the traditionally minded people in his department. At first he thought he might teach human gross anatomy using human fetuses, but that was not possible and he reverted to the use of cadavers. Dr. Robertson transformed gross anatomy for the medical students by recruiting four physical anthropologists to teach it.

Not all our new appointments worked as we had hoped. When we transformed radiology from a hospital unit to a full-fledged academic unit, I recruited Dick Lester to head the new Department of Radiology. He did well for the first few years, but he developed an enormous out-of-town schedule, so that he was out of Durham for twenty-eight days out of thirty, and the two days he was in town happened to be on the weekend, when he would come in to the office and dictate a whole stack of letters. I confronted him with this, and we agreed that the best thing he could do was to resign. He went on to positions elsewhere that he enjoyed more than he did running the Department of Radiology at Duke.

Around 1966 I had to persuade Jerry Harris to relinquish the chair in pediatrics. He was not recruiting or retaining outstanding people, and the Department of Pediatrics was beginning to slip. The search committee selected Sam Katz from Boston Children's Hospital. Sam had been a pioneer working with John Enders on the basic research that led to the development of the polio vaccine (Enders subsequently received the Nobel Prize for this work). Everybody told me about the numerous chairs Sam Katz had been offered, but all agreed that his family was determined to stay in Boston in perpetuity and that we would never get him. As it turned out, we did get him, and he did extremely well. Katz subsequently married Catherine Wilfert, also in Duke's Department of Pediatrics, who has done outstanding work in the research and treatment of pediatric AIDS.

In the mid-sixties, we determined that we needed some leadership in ophthalmology following the retirement of Banks Anderson Sr. The lead candidate for the position ended up being Joseph A. C. Wadsworth, who was a clinical professor of ophthalmology at Columbia University, with private offices on Park Avenue in New York. Joe had grown up in Durham and was very good friends with many of the leaders of the community; it turned out that he was also a close friend of Wright Tisdale, general counsel of the Ford Motor Company and chairman of the Duke University Board of Trustees.

Tisdale called Duke president Doug Knight to suggest that Joe Wadsworth be considered for the new chair in ophthalmology. President Knight called me, and I had no objection to having Dr. Wadsworth as the lead candidate, as he had all the credentials to be a leader in clinical ophthalmology, although there was no research component in his career. It was my judgment that this new, small department needed as its highest priority to develop its clinical base and to look at a subsequent generation for leadership in research. So we courted Joe Wadsworth. It was an easy courtship. It didn't take anything to persuade him to come back home to Durham, away from all the hoopla of life in New York City. Part of the agreement with Joe was that we build a new eye center, since the department was crammed into small quarters in the Davison Building. Joe did a good job of raising the money for the new eye center as well as in recruiting new and younger faculty.

When the time came for Joe's retirement, however, he was not very co-operative; I believe he thought he could stay on forever, which is not un-usual among people of retirement age. He was also upset that, in Duke's tradition, rather than naming the Eye Center the Wadsworth Eye Center in his honor, the building it was housed in would be called the Wadsworth Building. He was also quite irritated and negative about my appointment of Robert Machemer as his successor. Dr. Machemer was selected after a group of us visited both the Eye Center at Johns Hopkins and the Bascom-Palmer Institute at the University of Miami where Dr. Machemer was on the faculty. Dr. Machemer had opened up an entirely new frontier in sur-gery in the vitreous chamber, which had been a no-man's-land for ophthal-mology. All of the difficulties with Dr. Wadsworth eventually settled down, and Dr. Machemer built the next outstanding layer in ophthalmology, in-cluding a new research component. (Subsequently David Epstein, who has continued to do an outstanding job leading the ophthalmology faculty, succeeded him.)

The chair in the Department of Medicine became another bone of con-tention after Jim Wyngaarden was lured to Washington to become direc-tor of the NIH in 1982. (When Jim Wyngaarden was being considered for the directorship of the NIH, one sticking point by the powers in the White House under President Reagan was that Jim was a registered Democrat in Durham since his arrival in the mid-fifties. My explanation, which was ap-parently accepted, was that at the time one did not have a choice because the Republican Party was totally undeveloped in our community.)

We appointed a search committee to replace Wyngaarden, and one of the top candidates was Bill Kelley, until recently vice president of the Univer-sity of Pennsylvania and dean of its medical school. At that time, Dr. Kelley headed the Department of Medicine at the University of Michigan. He had trained at Duke, and I was always very impressed with his abilities. He was rather keen to come back. When I met with him, he had twelve demands, ten of which were far out of the ballpark of feasibility; and therefore, with the concurrence of other key department chairmen, I bade him farewell. Before Dr. Kelley, we had also looked at Bob Schrier, who chose to re-main chairman of medicine at the University of Colorado. He decided not to come to Duke because he and his family loved living in Denver. In the course of all of these events, Joe Greenfield, who had disqualified himself as being uninterested in the chair, came back to see me to say that after being subjected to interviews with other candidates, he felt he himself was a better candidate and he would like to go back in the competition. I presented this to the search committee and to MedSAC and got their concurrence to appoint Joe Greenfield chair of medicine.

Dr. Buettner-Janusch was one of the physical anthropologists we had recruited to teach gross anatomy under Dr. David Robertson. He had run into Phil Handler at the Denver airport and had managed to relate to Phil that he was unhappy at Yale where he had, as it happened, a primate colony of lemurs housed in the attic of the same old biology building where I grew up. Handler reported his conversation to me, and I seized the first opportunity of a trip to New Haven to interview Buettner-Janusch and persuade him to come to Duke—with his lemurs—which he did in 1965. I had to discuss this move with Taylor Cole, the provost of the university, since a primate colony was outside the sphere of responsibility of the Medical School, and, while I was happy to place Dr. Buettner-Janusch and other physical anthropologists on a full-time faculty salary, I did not want the responsibility for the budget and space of the primate center. So the primate colony became part of the university, the Duke Primate Center become world-famous, and Buettner-Janusch became one of the physical anthropologists who made gross anatomy such a popular course among the medical students. Year after year, several of these anthropologists won best-teaching awards from the Medical School.

Buettner-Janusch was also a problem, however, in that he would spend his weekends dictating multipage letters of complaint to the provost of the university, with copies to me. I remember in particular when Bill Bevan was provost: Bevan was so conscientious that he would respond to the letters item by item, writing multipage responses. Personally, I regarded the dictating machine as Buettner-Janusch's psychiatrist, a means of unloading his feelings on the weekends; I would send a very short note thanking him for relaying to me his ideas and his opinions. Ironically, we would meet on the grounds or in the hallways the next day, and he would thank me profusely for responding.

Subsequently, Buettner-Janusch got sufficiently annoyed with Duke that he moved to New York University, where he ran into one problem after another. For a while, his wife was able to keep him on the straight and narrow, but after she died, he went to pot, in more ways than one. He spent a good deal of time in the federal penitentiary for making illicit drugs in his laboratory. On being paroled, he made the mistake of sending chocolate candies laced with poison to the judge's wife. Fortunately, the ruse was discovered before she ate the candy, and in no time he was back in the penitentiary, where he died.

Another interesting but slightly embarrassing Duke faculty member was Walter Kempner. Dr. Kempner, a graduate of Heidelberg University School of Medicine, had become famous for treating various illnesses, including hypertension and diabetes, with a strict diet based on rice. When I first came to Duke in 1949, Dr. Kempner was a kingpin of the clinical practice. He was treated like a demigod, and nobody thought of doing anything except bowing low in his presence. He brought in a large income for the Department of Medicine, and his referrals to other specialists were an additional source of revenue. When I finished my residency in 1955, I was interested to note that Dr. Kempner was referring some of his private patients to me. Frequently these were women who had been extremely obese, and as they lost weight it became apparent that they had varicose veins and I would usually strip the veins. Dr. Kempner and I had a good professional relationship and were mutually respectful. Nobody actually befriended Dr. Kempner, and I do not know of anyone on the faculty—including Dr. Stead, the chief of his department—who had been invited to his home.

Kempner had two cars, which I understood were gifts from grateful patients. One was a Lincoln convertible, and the other was a Cadillac limousine. When it was raining, he used the Cadillac; when it was sunny, even though it might be freezing, he rode in his convertible with the top down and his bald head exposed to the air. Next to him would be two of his female assistants, and, when they were in the convertible they would be bundled up in every bit of fur clothing they could find. It was in these vehicles that he went from his office and clinic at Duke and to his various "rice houses."

My appearance in 1949 coincided with the year when sympathectomies were done to remove the sympathetic chains for hypertension, and the rice diet was gradually changing to a diet for morbidly obese people rather than for patients with hypertension, since antihypertensive drugs were coming into use.

In 1959, when my wife, Connie, and I were planning a trip to Rome, Ernest Peschel, who worked with Dr. Kempner, advised me that the only hotel to stay at in Rome was the Hassler, located at the top of the Spanish Steps. When we arrived at the Hassler, I saw Dr. Kempner, having an argument with the assistant manager across the registration desk; he was so engrossed in the argument that he did not see me. I was not very surprised to see Kempner. I had heard that he spent three months a year in Rome and Italy as part of his contract when he was recruited in the thirties by Dr. Frederic Hanes, then chairman of medicine. I went up to Dr. Kempner and tapped him on the shoulder. He swung around, saying, "Ach, mein Gott, what brings you here?" I said we were visiting the Vatican medical school. He asked who recommended the hotel, and I said, "Dr. Peschel" "And who do you think recommended it to Dr. Peschel?" he asked. "The great Walter Kempner himself," I replied. And he said, "Ach so, you are right." On future trips to Rome, particularly during the summertime, I would invariably see him either at the Hassler or going through the Vatican Museum.

During my tenure as head of the Medical Center, I began to do less and less surgery, so I no longer had professional contact with Dr. Kempner. It was not until the fall of 1972 that I had direct contact with him again. At a Saturday afternoon football game, Jim Wyngaarden, then chairman of medicine, sought me out and told me about an episode regarding Dr. Kempner. It seemed he had been whipping one of his patients in the medical PDC at Duke; he called it "aversive therapy" and administered it to patients who did not do his bidding. In consultation with Ken Pye, legal counsel for the university at the time, we decided to suspend Dr. Kempner from the Duke premises, pending further investigation. Jim Wyngaarden and I had the painful duty of informing Dr. Kempner of this decision. I do not believe that Dr. Kempner ever set foot on the premises after his suspension. He never forgave me.

On one occasion several years later, at the urging of Dr. Stead, I did go to visit Dr. Kempner at one of the rice houses on a social call, to see how he was getting along. I believe Dr. Stead's interest was mainly in seeing that Dr. Kempner would bequeath the Department of Medicine a major amount of money, but I did not get involved in that level of discussion with Dr. Kempner. Dr. Kempner saw my visit as one of apology, but it was not. By paying this short call, I was just trying to be humanitarian with an aging emeritus faculty member. I did not see Dr. Kempner on any of my subsequent travels, nor did I have anything further to do with him until a lawsuit was brought against him in the early nineties and I was deposed on my relationship with him. The lawsuit, brought on behalf of a young female patient, accused Dr. Kempner of subjecting her as well as other patients to "various abusive and improper procedures," including whippings and other objectionable activities. The case was settled and Kempner died subsequently.

In retrospect, I see Walter Kempner as a great individual who lost his way. He had been fortunate to escape Nazi Germany when he came to Duke in the thirties. He hit the peak of his career in the late thirties and forties, but began to go downhill probably in the late fifties and sixties, when his rice diet went from being the only source of treatment for malignant hypertension to one among several treatments for morbid obesity. The other diet programs in Durham owe much to Kempner's program; as matter of fact, Durham—and Duke—have become famous as home to a number of diet and lifestyle programs. What was unique about Walter Kempner is the fact that he was extremely strict and Germanic with his patients. It was not unusual to hear him say to a patient, "You will do this or you will die," which must have scared his patients into sticking with the rice diet. Some came back repeatedly to lose and relose their weight. The wife of a New Jersey governor, in her career as a patient several decades ago, probably lost a thousand pounds as the result of frequent visits.

While Dr. Kempner and Dr. Buettner-Janusch certainly helped make the Medical Center more interesting, they did not necessarily do great things for our reputation. But they were exceptions to the trend of continued change and growth for the better among the faculty as a whole.

By 1988, before I became chancellor of the University, Duke University Medical Center ranked number 3 in the listings of *U.S. News & World Report*. The only two ahead of us were Harvard and Hopkins, and I could see the justification for that ranking. Harvard is a large conglomerate, and Hopkins a renowned and long-established institution; both in the aggregate had much more NIH support than we did. It is a source of great pride to me that, during my tenure as dean, vice president, and chancellor of medical affairs, the Medical Center had risen from barely being on the map nationally to becoming one of the top academic medical centers in the nation.

6

CHANGING THE INSTITUTION

IMPROVING THE QUALITY and standing of the Duke hospital and Medical School was not just a matter of finding the right faculty to lead the departments. It also meant restructuring the institution, which included such measures as changing the way moneys were allocated, reorganizing and developing departments and programs, and bringing in the best administrators. Like any living organism, medical institutions change with the years, adapting to new conditions as these arise. And so, a number of institutional changes took place in my early years at the helm of the Medical Center.

In 1964 the very first problem meeting I had as a new dean was with the basic science chairmen. They had just received NIH funding for what is now the Nanaline Duke Building, and Vice Provost Woodhall had told them they would get a certain significant contribution from the PDC building fund toward the construction of that building. The PDC building fund was controlled by the clinical chairmen, but unfortunately Woodhall had neglected to tell the clinical chairmen about this commitment he had made on their behalf to the basic sciences. So there was a meeting at the house of Phil Handler, chairman of biochemistry, where all the basic science chairmen were gathered, and the meeting got to be a little bit heated. I didn't say a word because I didn't know the background, and it was fairly typical of Woodhall in such situations to just stomp out. So there I was, trying to figure out how I was going to make peace with this group of upset people. As it turned out, the clinical chairmen did agree to make the promised contribution. It took a bit of persuasion on my part, because up to that time, the PDC building fund went only toward clinical buildings. This was a major breakthrough that helped make Duke not only a better clinical center but a better medical center as a whole, with the clinical departments supporting the basic sciences.

Subsequently, I asked the PDCs to contribute about $800,000 to the Seeley G. Mudd Building, which houses the Medical Center library—after all, medical students and clinicians make use of this facility as much as any researcher, perhaps more so. My threat was that I would not approve of any other use of the building fund until that appropriation was made. I did not use muscle very often, but I could veto anything I wanted to. The PDCs in general had their own organization, headed by the chairmen of the clinical departments, and I would leave them alone to function as they saw fit, except when I had an interest, as with the Seeley G. Mudd Building, in having a major contribution to the Medical Center in general.

The PDCs also contributed $5 million toward the equity of the new hospital, with another $5 million coming from their departmental funds ($2 million each from surgery and medicine, and the remaining $1 million allocated in the proportions in which they contributed to the building fund per se), so that the clinical departments ended up giving $10 million toward the $40 million in equity of the new hospital. This made it easier for me to persuade The Duke Endowment to match that with another $10 million, given over a seven-year period, as well as to attract other donors. Under Dr. Davison, the clinical departments had kept the basic sciences at arm's length, but with these decisions, the two parts of the Medical Center came to function as one unit within the larger structure of the university.

The PDC building fund was also used to recruit chairmen. Originally this was limited to clinical chairmen, but I got it changed to help with the recruitment of all chairmen, with a lump sum available for the kind of fiscal enticement sometimes needed to bring in new people. It has been very helpful in that regard. The clinical chairmen recognized that their basic strength in research depended on the quality of the basic science departments and their graduate programs.

In 1964 the financial books of the PDCs were not available for the dean to see. Despite the fact that Dr. Hart, former chairman of surgery, was the immediate past president of the university and Dr. Stead, chairman of medicine, was a force to contend with, I insisted that the books be under the purview of the dean and, ultimately, of the Duke University Board of Trustees. With the help of Henry Rauch, one of our financially most astute trustees, we set up the ground rules for the university overview of the operations of the PDCs. It took a few years of negotiations between the university lawyers and the PDC lawyers, but the result was that the annual audit of the PDCs would be made available in a one-page summary to the executive committee of the trustees. The full audit would be given to me as well as to appropriate members of the university and Medical Center administrations.

Then there was the question of salaries. I insisted that all salaries be known to me, as dean of the school, and that no negotiations of faculty salaries should go forward without my knowing of it. In 1930–32, when Dr. Hart and Dr. Davison had agreed on the formation of the PDCs, the contribution of the Medical School budget to an individual physician's salary was only $2,500. By the time I became dean in 1964, the clinical faculty were still only getting $2,500 from the university budget, and the rest of the salary, whether it was $30,000 or $40,000, came from the pooled clinical earnings of the faculty. (The pooled earnings were separate from the building fund, which took 8 percent off the top of the PDC income before it went to the various departments for their reserves.) As the sixties and early seventies went along, it became apparent that the clinical faculty was missing out on fringe benefits such as the retirement fund. With the concurrence of the clinical chairmen we therefore stepped up the amount of money that came through the university by recirculating the clinical money. So a professor's salary would consist of four layers: a base layer from the pooled PDC income, $2,500 from the original university endowment contribution through the Medical Center budget; fringe benefits paid out of recirculated clinical department funds; and finally, an amount that the department paid the clinical faculty member to attract and retain that person. So, for example, an associate professor's salary of $40,000 would comprise $2,500 from the Medical School budget and $37,500 from recirculated clinical department funds; on top of that $40,000 he or she would get fringe benefits and a direct payment from the PDC, making the total salary package competitive with the market.

Basic science faculty got their full salary through the university, although maximum benefit was derived from research grants; we made sure that researchers put down a permissible percentage of their time and salary to come from that grant. Of course, the problem is deciding how much soft money to build into the system to forestall such potential crises as having the NIH budget torpedoed in any given year. Once tenure is given to a basic science faculty member, the Medical School and university are responsible for sustaining that salary. This became something of a problem when some of the basic science faculty got older and were no longer competitive with

NIH or NSF granting. We were very careful not to let that get out of hand, and of course I depended in good measure on the appropriate department chairmen to help monitor the situation.

Tenure is a time-honored custom whereby an academic is assured a permanent position on the faculty if he or she fulfills certain requirements in a satisfactory manner over a set probationary period, traditionally seven years. One of the main arguments in favor of tenure has always been that it gives academics the freedom to act and speak according to their consciences, even if the opinions are unpopular at the time. One of the main arguments against it is that many people, once they have acquired tenure, sink into a comfortable semiretirement—no need to knock yourself out publishing or doing research, because you can't be fired. Academics cling to tenure with great tenacity, even though we are no longer talking of academic life in the Middle Ages, when tenure was a very valuable concept.

Tenure at the Medical Center was modified after 1964. First, we developed a track for medical research professors, whereby the individual would not receive university tenure and his or her salary was contingent on the availability of research funding. I had always advocated something different; namely, to abolish tenure and institute five-year roll-forward funding, but I could never sell it to the university administration or to the Academic Council (the representative body of the entire university faculty). It never moved to the front burner because all the signals I got were that it would not fly.

Instead, it took me about four years to work through the Academic Council the idea of prolonging the period of consideration of tenure in the Medical School from seven years to eleven years. If you are going to grant—or deny—tenure within seven years, you have to decide within five and a half years whether to initiate the process to get people tenure or to prepare them to leave the institution. This seemed like too short a period in which to consider a lifetime obligation to a medical faculty member. That is why we stretched it to eleven years, even though the wording in the agreement with the Academic Council and the university was that the individual departments would have to vote on it. This was not particularly a problem with the clinical departments. As we looked at the matter, it turned out that different components of the university have quite different views on tenure. Apparently the Law School makes a tenure decision around the third year, which is, I gather, the way of life in law schools around the country. But it certainly would be too short a period for the basic medical sciences.

Drawing the clinical departments and basic sciences together and rationalizing the process for salary decisions and tenure were two crucial elements in the restructuring of the Medical Center. There were also some difficult decisions to be made about some of the institution's programs: the Nursing School, the Program in Health Administration, and the various specialty centers that were founded in this period.

I have always been a strong supporter of the nursing profession. Even as a young faculty member in the Department of Surgery, I was involved to a minor extent in the education of some of the nursing students in the master's degree program. They came to my fourth-year surgical outpatient conferences and sat with the medical students, and some of the nursing students could answer my questions just as well as if not better than the medical students. At that time I also befriended Ruby Wilson, a nursing clinical instructor, whom I hired subsequently as dean of the School of Nursing.

My first experience with the School of Nursing when I became dean was with Ann Jacobansky, who had run the diploma program in nursing and had put it through its subsequent transformation into a baccalaureate program. She was very easy to work with, and we got along fine. After her retirement, a university committee headed by Frank deVyver, the assistant provost, looked for a successor and ended up with Myrtle Irene Brown from the University of Missouri. I tried to work with Dr. Brown as a full-fledged colleague of equal rank, but she was a very difficult person. She had persuaded Dr. Woodhall to have her housemate, who had retired from the army, appointed chief of the nursing service at Duke Hospital. Together, the chief of the nursing service and the dean caused a fair amount of difficulty. One night they announced to me, without any notice whatsoever, that they would close one-third of the hospital beds within days on the basis of maintaining the quality of care. The big mistake they made was to have a press conference before they came to see me. I put the director of nursing services on leave of absence with pay, and appointed a committee, headed by Dr. Parker of ob-gyn and Wilma Minnear of the nursing faculty, to investigate what had gone wrong. At the conclusion of that investigation, we terminated the director of nursing services and I persuaded Miss Minnear to shed her academic cloak and take on the position of director of nursing services, which she filled admirably for many years. In the meantime, things became more and more disagreeable with Dean Brown, and, with the help of the provost of the university, Dr. Marcus Hobbs, we were able to get her to resign. I then invited Ruby Wilson to assume the leadership of the School of Nursing.

Shortly after this, Chancellor Kenneth Pye of the university issued his retrenchment study, in which he pointed out that we could not do every-thing we were doing and maintain quality standards. One of the areas he felt we should close down was the entire School of Nursing. I used up most of my brownie points with the university leadership in persuading them to let us retain the graduate master's program in a new form: we would edu-cate clinical nursing leaders rather than the sociologic types that had been produced in the past. But I could not defend the undergraduate program, in which many of the matriculants had SAT and grade point averages below those of the other students admitted as undergraduates by the university. In the course of this transition, I received many bullets from nurses and nurs-ing education leaders from all over the country; they did not appreciate the fine distinction between the role that I played retaining a graduate program versus what the university wanted to do. But it all ended up well, in that the graduate program in nursing has been thriving under the leadership of Dean Mary Champagne, and now has something close to two hundred stu-dents who are mostly part-time students or part-time staff (the part-time staff get a 90 percent remission in tuition). They end up as leaders in clinical nursing.

When I took over in 1964, very few programs in the Medical Center were coordinated or driven from a central base. Each department was pretty much on its own. An example of one of the earliest ways to unify the in-stitution was the construction in the early seventies of the Medical Center library as a resource that would serve everybody—premed student, Ph.D. candidate, post-doc, resident, or faculty—as a central resource. This move was resisted by some of the larger departments, which did not want to see Medical Center building fund money going toward matching money raised for the Medical Center library.

The effort to do things across the board emerged only gradually in my time. The new hospital was instrumental in that respect, as was the emer-gence of the various "centers" in the seventies. These centers have not only crossed departmental lines in the clinical sciences but have also dipped into the basic sciences in their all-encompassing missions.

As a result of President Nixon's determination to wage a "war on can-cer," the National Cancer Institute put out an all-points bulletin inviting academic institutions to submit proposals for the establishment of cancer centers. We were very fortunate at Duke in 1972 to have some very strong cancer researchers, and with the leadership of Dr. William Shingleton in general surgery, Dr. Wayne Rundles in medicine, and Wolfgang Joklik in microbiology and immunology, we presented a plan that gave Duke one of the first comprehensive cancer centers in the country. "Comprehensive" referred to the fact that it combined equally important interdepartmental programs in clinical care and research. The center leadership managed to assemble boards of visitors and consultants who were really outstanding, and who did a lot of very successful fundraising, which continues to this day.

The Duke Heart Center, which was established later on, has lagged in that regard. Interestingly, it was more difficult teasing heart research support and facilities out of the control of the traditional departments than it had been to establish the Cancer Center. To this day, the Cancer Center is more fully developed and more semiautonomous than the Heart Center. Part of the reason is that people like Dr. Sabiston, in surgery, did not see any benefit in having a separate component as a heart center with separate budget and space since it duplicated a main thrust of the general and thoracic program at Duke. I could appreciate Dr. Sabiston's traditional view. In medicine, the key figure at that time was probably Andy Wallace, and I don't recall that we had a strong push from him either to establish a heart center, other than as a loosely knit amalgam of the efforts going on in the heart field. Later, however, with Jerry Reeves, probably one of the world's outstanding cardiac anesthesiologists (and now with Tom Ryan), the center began to pick up pace.

The advantages of having these separate centers is for fundraising and for obtaining grants from the National Cancer Institute or the Heart/Lung Institute of the NIH, or the American Heart Association or American Cancer Society. However, there is a benign conflict of interest in academic medical centers. Do you lop off the space and the budget that pertain to cancer or heart research, and have vertical components in cancer or heart? Or do you maintain the horizontal components of surgery that include heart surgery and of medicine that includes oncology? These are things that each generation of chairmen and leaders of the centers needs to work out.

The potential for conflict is not only among the leadership, but also at the level of the development staffs. The development staff of the centers keep bumping into other development staffs trying to respond to the needs of the academic departments. Then there are the other centers, like the Children's Center, which deals with all the problems of children including cancer and heart disease; the Nutrition Center; the Eye Center—and on and on. In every university there is this tension in fund-raising as to who gets first dibs on a potential donor or a foundation supporting this or that field. Clearly in a university the president has to make the decision between the medical center and other components of the university. Within the medical center, it has to be left to the office of the chancellor for health affairs (or its equivalent) to make the decision. What you do not want is to have two groups of individuals soliciting from a major donor simultaneously. That can be very embarrassing—and it has happened.

The Veterans Administration has been a very important component of the total Medical Center in that it has provided patients to be cared for by the resident staff, under the supervision of faculty who have joint appointments at Duke and the VA. I do not know the precise figures on how the population and epidemiology have changed in the past ten years; my impression is that, as everywhere in the practice of medicine, the VA has become more outpatient-oriented. It is interesting that when the VA opened its doors in 1953, it was against the law to see anyone there as an outpatient—there was no such term in the VA vocabulary. Outpatients were smuggled in under the label NBO ("nonbed occupant") and seen in the doctors' examining rooms on the various wards because there was no outpatient clinic. Now there are some VA facilities, such as one in South Florida, that are geared exclusively to outpatient care. (In 1964, when I was a new dean visiting the VA headquarters in Washington, I suggested to Dr. Joseph McNinch, the chief medical director, that the VA consider becoming an insurance agency rather than a health care system that could not compete with the academic medical centers. Veterans with wartime injuries and their dependents would be covered for 100 percent of their care; others would pay on a sliding scale. Fortunately, McNinch and his staff did not take the suggestion seriously, and now the VA system is a tremendous asset to the health care of veterans and to the medical education and research programs of the nation.)

An institution's buildings or programs may be well conceived and initiated, but they will not perform well if they are not managed well. People make the difference. So we worked assiduously at recruiting and retaining the best support staff, and in some cases, to let those who were not successful move on. By the late sixties, it had become more and more apparent that Charlie Frenzel, the lay administrator of Duke Hospital, could no longer function well in that capacity. As a man without an M.D., he was at a severe disadvantage in making major decisions that affected the powerhouse of clinical chairmen whom I had recruited. About the same time, Stuart Sessoms was finishing up his tour of duty as deputy director to James Shannon at the NIH. He was looking for a job in the private sector. I contacted our alumnus Marty Cummings, director of the National Library of Medicine, who was a close personal friend of the Sessoms family. He encouraged me to pursue Stuart. In any event, I thought it would be great to have an M.D., who had been trained to make major decisions, come and be in charge of the hospital, and so Stuart Sessoms succeeded Charlie Frenzel.

For several years, Stuart functioned very well in relating to the clinical chairmen. Obviously they had some concerns about Stuart diluting their authority, but they went along with the appointment, and Stuart was low-key enough that he did not seem to be threatening. Unfortunately, toward the end of Stuart's directorship he tended to come to my office every day in the late afternoon to run the problems of the day by me. This was contrary to the way in which I had learned to delegate authority: I always told the people I recruited that I would expect them to make 95 percent of the decisions in their various areas on their own but use their judgment in bringing the remaining 5 percent of their problems to my attention. Likewise, if I had reason to bring something to their attention, I would do so within that 5 percent margin. So when Stuart started bringing all of his problems by on a daily basis, I started getting somewhat sharp and critical with him. Nevertheless, he surprised me one Thanksgiving when I was at Beech Mountain: he called me up and told me that he was resigning to take the job as the number 2 person at Blue Cross/Blue Shield of North Carolina. He had not given me any indication that this was in the offing, though clearly he had been negotiating with them for some time. This was a bitter pill, but as I reflected on it, I thought maybe it was for the best. As the Arabs would say when I was growing up, "It is God's will." In his separation letter he asked to be paid for all the sick and vacation days that he had not taken. I did not dispute the fact and had him paid what I considered an atrocious request, but it was the price of being able to find a new leader of the hospital.

One of the prime candidates to succeed Sessoms was Dr. Roscoe R. Robinson, better known as Ike. I was interested in promoting someone from the inside since we were at a critical juncture, about to build a major new hospital, and I did not want to take the time to educate somebody from scratch. Dr. Robinson had come to Duke as an intern in 1954 and had moved up through the ranks; when the hospital directorship opened once again, Ike had been chief of nephrology for many years and had achieved international recognition for his leadership in this specialty. He had climbed all the mountains that could be climbed as a nephrologist. So it seemed an opportune time for him to consider a career where he did not have to give up nephrology but would devote the greater part of his time to running Duke University Hospital and to help with planning the new North Division of that hospital. Ike, always diligent, called Stuart, who apparently was quite derogatory about any working relationship with me. Nevertheless, in his wisdom, Ike accepted the job of CEO of the hospital in 1976 while retaining his position as chief of the division of nephrology. He was in that position for five years. He was a very good peacemaker, a good listener, a good person to patch things up. I valued his advice and followed it fairly closely.

Ike had also not given up on being available as a candidate for other important jobs in the country. Up to that time, he had looked at chairmanships in various departments of medicine. When he was offered the opportunity to become my equivalent at Vanderbilt University—with the title there of "vice chancellor," since the chancellor is the head of the university—I encouraged him to take it, in spite of the loss this represented for Duke. So in 1981 Ike went to Vanderbilt, where he has done an outstanding job of rebuilding their medical center. Ike and his wife, Ann, were good leaders not just at Duke, but also in the greater Durham community.

When Ike accepted the job as head of Duke Hospital, he had one stipulation: that he be able to move Bill Donelan, then assistant to the chairman of medicine, to be his chief business and financial officer in the hospital. When Ike left, Bill stayed on and worked extremely well with Ike's successor, Dr. Andrew Wallace. They formed a good team. Subsequently, Bill has done an outstanding job as the chief financial and business officer for the Duke University Medical Center and, as it is now known, the Duke University Health System.

After Ike's departure, I had asked again for candidates and was presented with the possibility of enticing Andy Wallace to the position of director of Duke hospital. Andy had been chief of cardiology at Duke at the age of thirty-five, a very young age for such a post, and, like Ike Robinson, he had achieved the summit in his chosen field. He had introduced a rehabilitation program for cardiology patients, and as an outgrowth of that, he was instrumental in establishing the Center for Living, a large, very successful program that helps people with cardiovascular disease or at risk for heart disease to learn and follow healthy lifestyles (the clinic building in the Center for Living is named for him). He had also done important research. Andy was a recognized national leader among other groups such as the Markle scholars. Whatever Andy did, he did extremely well. Like Ike, he also had a great partner, his wife, Barrie, who was active in Durham and Duke affairs.

Andy was the person I thought I was grooming to be my successor when the day of my retirement came along. In 1988, when I accepted the move to the Allen Building as chancellor of Duke University, I honestly felt that Andy Wallace was the best qualified person to succeed me as executive vice president and chancellor for health affairs at Duke University. However, it became apparent that he and Keith Brodie, who was then the university president, did not get along. Looking into the matter subsequently, I gathered that when Andy was director of the hospital and Keith was chairman of psychiatry, Keith had appeared one day in Andy's office with some demand that Andy had denied. Apparently, Brodie never forgave him. I was not aware of that at the time. Keith appointed a search committee to look for my successor and although they interviewed Andy, he was not chosen for the position. I had seen similar turns in other university medical centers, when personal animosities and loyalties had changed the direction of an individual's career and often, as a result, that of an institution. I had made many changes in restructuring the Duke Medical Center, but in the end, was not able to pass the baton on to one of our most able people. In 1990 Andy became dean of the Dartmouth medical school and vice president for health affairs of Dartmouth College, where he has done an outstanding job.

7

TRANSFORMING MEDICAL
EDUCATION

WHEN DUKE MEDICAL SCHOOL began in 1930, the curriculum to a large degree followed the Hopkins pattern, which in turn was influenced by Abraham Flexner's influential report of 1910 on medical education in the United States and Canada. Much of the curriculum was elective: only 54 percent of the hours were allotted to required courses. But then came medical progress, and with it, more and more knowledge that was considered essential. Elective courses gave way to required ones, so that the students' heads could be filled with all the knowledge they would need to be successful practitioners for the next thirty to thirty-five years. By 1955 a visitor from the Commonwealth Fund noted that the Duke Medical School's "four-year program amounts to 5,148 teaching hours of which only 17 are free time. This is really tight!" In practice, this meant overtaxed students, who saw the amount of knowledge they had to acquire continually exceeding the time available for learning, while also making it very difficult to explore special interests in a time when specialization was the growing trend.

In 1955–56 the faculty spent considerable time discussing this problem. Especially involved were Philip Handler and Gene Stead. Handler, the biochemist, saw that the availability of funding after World War II made possible great increases in medical research but the educational process did not provide for a concomitant rise in the number of people who could function as both clinicians and researchers. He saw a particular need for increasing the number of basic researchers. He proposed taking a number of exceptional students after two years of medical school and giving them nine months of intensive training in a basic discipline, under the guidance of specialists in the various fields. By taking additional classes during two summers, the students could complete their medical training with their classmates. Handler hoped that out of each group of eighteen students, five or six would choose to finish a Ph.D. in a basic discipline, as well as the M.D., and thus add to the needed pool of teachers and researchers in either clinical medicine or preclinical science.

This proposal became the start of the Research Training Program (RTP), which evolved into a fifteen-month unit that could be inserted into the Medical School curriculum and also into the residency programs of the clinical services to train people in fundamental basic research. Philip Handler secured the funding for the program and asked Dr. James Wyngaarden if he was interested in heading it—which he did, working with Monte Moses, Sam Gross, Joe Blum, Saleh Wakil, and others who had followed him from Washington University in Saint Louis. Both Dr. Hart and Dr. Stead agreed to let students spend one academic quarter in the RTP as a substitute for one of the two required quarters in each of medicine and surgery. Stead was particularly enthusiastic about the program. He was—and still is—a firm believer in establishing patterns of curiosity that will lead a student to a lifetime of learning, and he saw the RTP as an excellent step in that direction. The basic science experience could tie in with a clinical interest the student already wanted to pursue—or, for that matter, be in an entirely different area, opening new fields of interest.

The only criticism came from the medical students the RTP was intended to serve, who wanted the chance to experience some clinical work before spending a year in research. So the program was modified to be open to students after the third year of medical school.

The RTP was set up for both medical students and residents, primarily residents in medicine and in pediatrics, and was the only program for training residents to become clinician-scientists until I started the Surgical Scholars Program. I had happened to attend an American College of Surgeons surgical forum session in 1961, where it dawned on me that the papers being presented by surgical residents were purely mechanical. They were finding new ways to hook up one piece of gut to the other, but that was not basic research. So I talked with Jim Wyngaarden and Phil Handler, and we started a program whereby early in the residency, a surgical resident could take time out for the RTP course; we would protect a certain amount of his or her time in the ensuing several years so that he or she could maintain the research program. We applied and received NIH support for the Surgical

Scholars Program. When Dr. Sabiston came in 1964, he took it over and expanded it to a very successful program.

While all this was taking place, the study that Barnes Woodhall had commissioned from the consultancy firm Booz, Allen & Hamilton was presented. It emphasized the need not only for physical change on the Medical Center campus but for programmatic change as well. They, too, saw the need for strengthening the teaching of the basic sciences and for educating basic as well as clinical scientists. At about this time, as Dr. Wyngaarden remembers it, Handler, Tosteson, Stead, and Jerome Harris, the chairman of pediatrics (who was also a biochemist), were having lunch one day, when Tosteson said, "If that [RTP] program is good for six students a year, why not sixty?" And thus the idea for a new curriculum for the M.D. program— a return, in a sense, to the old curriculum—was born.

In 1959, after Dr. Wiley Forbus, the original chair in pathology, retired, Dr. Thomas B. Kinney was recruited by Duke from Case Western Reserve in Cleveland. He brought with him the experience of a new curriculum introduced at Western Reserve around 1956. The one thing that his Western Reserve experience showed was that significant changes could be made in the curriculum, and it could be done without losing faculty. Western Reserve did not have a core curriculum. Instead, they took what was taught vertically and coordinated it horizontally by system. With the cardiovascular system, for instance, instead of medicine and surgery teaching about the heart separately, it was coordinated across the board. Dr. Herbert Sieker, a young faculty member in medicine, was appointed chairman of the new curriculum committee and oversaw all the discussions and faculty retreats focused on educational change.

Duke's "new curriculum," as it finally evolved, consisted of two years of "core" courses and two years of electives. In the first year of medical school, a basic core curriculum is taught in the basic sciences—anatomy, biochemistry, physiology, neurological sciences, genetics, pathology, microbiology, and pharmacology. The second year brings in a clinical science core curriculum in medicine, surgery, obstetrics, pediatrics, and psychiatry. These two years are carefully structured to give the student the rudiments— above all, a knowledge of the vocabulary—on which he or she can build. The remaining two years are elective: the third year brings deeper exploration in the basic sciences, while the fourth year brings greater experience in the clinical area or areas that the student intends to pursue.

Interestingly, while the new curriculum gave students the option of spending the entire third year in one or two areas in the basic medical sciences, as it turned out, only about 25 percent chose that option. The rest of the students took a smorgasbord of subjects that are probably bridge areas between the clinical and the basic sciences. The real potential academicians have been the students who elect the M.D.-Ph.D. course. In retrospect, I see that it really takes at least three years of careful nurturing of research skills to become an investigator who can command support from agencies such as the NIH.

The Duke Medical School owes its tradition of flexibility and adaptability first to Dr. Davison. When he was an undergraduate at Princeton, he wanted to quit after two years and go immediately to Columbia Physicians and Surgeons Medical School, but his father, who was a rather stern taskmaster, insisted that he finish Princeton first. When he finished in 1913, he was named a Rhodes scholar, and the first thing he did when he arrived in Oxford was to knock on the door of Sir William Osler's residence and ask whether he could compress his two years of medical study into one; he was looking for flexibility and ways to trim things here and there. "Here comes yet another American colt trying to change Oxford tradition," was Dr. Osler's comment to his wife. But Davison was very fluid and adaptable. He certainly came to Duke with a flexible, open mind. Gene Stead also came to Duke willing to change traditional approaches. I well remember his admonition that we should teach students how to learn, rather than teach them what we, as teachers, wanted them to learn.

From 1963 onward Dr. Woodhall and I convened periodic retreats for the faculty. It was essential that the faculty be on board for the changes, because it meant a great readjustment for most of them. Each department had to decide what knowledge was truly vital and how to convey this knowledge most effectively. Most departments lost teaching hours. Obviously, small-group teaching and a great deal of supervision were needed to make the program work. It was apparent when we were looking at the new curriculum in 1964, with the hope of putting it in full swing in 1966, that we were going to need some pump-priming money other than what we had in the operating budget of the Medical School. It was at that point that I approached the Commonwealth Fund of New York for a major five-year grant of $750,000 to support the changes. Lester Evans was the vice president of the fund at that time, and I can still remember the joy I felt when he called me one evening to let me know that the Commonwealth Fund had approved what they considered the largest grant they had ever given to help us with the new curriculum

The intent of the new curriculum at Duke was to avoid cramming into four years all the facts that the medical student would need for a lifetime of practice; it was an acknowledgment that only 50 percent of the facts of the day would still be valid five years later, and that there was a continuing change in the facts of medicine relating to the practice of medicine. Our emphasis in the new curriculum was on learning to learn for a lifetime, and that it was not a cause for shame not to know a certain fact, because it could be looked up. In my own rounds in surgery with the students and the resident staff—on an average of once a week with the residents and with the students for a semester each year—I would make it a point to respond to some questions, "I don't know the answer, why don't we look it up together and come back with a report to the group?" An alumna who graduated from Duke twenty years ago told me that the one thing she learned from me was not to be embarrassed to say, "I don't know."

From 1961 to 1975 the number of applications to Duke rose 652 percent, with greater geographical diversity than we had had before. Class sizes gradually grew from about 60 to 110. Medical schools from across the country showed an interest in the curricular changes, and visitors were most enthusiastic at what they saw.

The Medical School did not rest at changing just the M.D. curriculum and instituting the RTP and Surgical Scholars Program. It also took a harder look at its training of clinician-scientists. The program that it had in place, the Research Training Program, was a fifteen-month unit that could be inserted into the Medical School curriculum and also into the residency programs of the clinical services to train people in fundamental basic research. In the sixties it became apparent that the two research programs were not sufficient. So, with support from the National Institute of General Medical Sciences (NIGMS), the M.D.-Ph.D. program was conceived, which gives students three full years of training in research after the complete core medical curriculum, followed by one final clinical year. Tom Kinney, a member of the council of the NIGMS, helped pioneer the development of the M.D.-Ph.D. program nationally as well as at Duke. It was also a dream of Jim Shannon's, then head of the NIH, to educate a generation of people with a foot in each camp, in basic science and in clinical medicine.

Duke was one of the first three institutions to receive funding for an M.D.-Ph.D. program. Today there are fifty or sixty such programs. To the chagrin of those who see a need for more clinical investigators, however, the M.D.-Ph.D. programs have not produced them. The primary product has been bench scientists with medical school backgrounds. Most graduates go into cell biology, although at Duke an unusually high percentage have gone into pathology, thanks to the influence of Tom Kinney. It has also produced a fortunate group of debt-free scientists, since NIH supports the programs handsomely with stipends and tuition grants. As the M.D.-Ph.D. program took hold at Duke, the Research Training Program phased out, especially since the NIH did not want to support two such expensive programs. The Surgical Scholars Program was also discontinued, in 1993, for the same reasons.

The need for clinical investigators continues. Over the last sixty years, three levels of research have evolved. First, there is the clinical investigation of patients that is now conducted on a global scale, where you have physicians and nurses monitoring various types of therapy that are standardized centrally. This kind of clinical research is more apt to be supported by pharmaceutical companies than the NIH. Second, there is the more fundamental kind of clinical research, which does not directly investigate humans and which is supported by the NIH and the NSF—particularly the NIH. Finally, there is fundamental basic research, unrelated to a specific illness, which is conducted today either by Ph.D.'s in the basic medical sciences or by M.D.-Ph.D.'s working in the style of basic scientists.

In 1979, during the time he was chairman of medicine at Duke, Jim Wyngaarden wrote an article titled "The Clinical Investigator as an Endangered Species," which appeared in the *New England Journal of Medicine*. The gist of his argument was that clinical researchers—trained in both fundamental biomedical research and clinical medicine—were a dying breed. The article was, and is, much quoted around the country. It was the first time that people woke up to the fact that NIH funding was drifting either to Ph.D.'s or to full-time researchers, but that clinical investigators with a foot in each camp—that is, clinical medicine and basic research—were receiving a decreasing amount of the NIH money. The M.D.-Ph.D. program that started at Duke in the 1960s aimed to compensate for this lack of robustness in the research capabilities of clinicians, but the problem is an ongoing one. It has become clear that you would have a difficult time today being a good clinician (one I would want to take care of me) and still be a researcher of Nobel quality. In most academic medical centers, particularly private institutions, anybody spending a significant amount of time on research rather than patient care needs to keep getting NIH grants. With 20 percent or less of approved grants being funded, the competition is intense, and the people getting hotly contested funding have very little time to do clinical work to maintain their clinical proficiency.

The leadership at Duke Medical Center did not try to guide individual research from a central position; it was left mainly to the individual departments. For most of my years, the Department of Medicine had the largest NIH support of any department, basic or clinical, in the institution. This was especially true in the heydays of Drs. Stead and Wyngaarden, and to some extent with Dr. Greenfield. The Department of Medicine continues to be the largest recipient of NIH funds of any department in the school. The department, which used to be ranked in the top five in NIH funding in the nation, dropped out of the top ten for several years; however, it climbed back to number 10 in the rankings in 1999, a major feat, accomplished by its chair, Dr. Barton Haynes.

When Dr. Carl Chapman was president of the Commonwealth Fund in the late seventies, he asked me along with two or three other people to meet him at the fund's offices in New York City to discuss what else the fund should do to innovate medical education. I proposed that we start an interface program between the Medical School and the university, so that we could link up with undergraduate students, giving them access to the Medical School's basic science courses as well as showing them the care delivery side of the Medical School. I mentioned this particular program in 1976 to the Medical School advisory committee at Duke and said that we were preparing a grant proposal that Dr. Chapman had invited us to submit for that purpose. At that time, Dr. Tosteson was professor of physiology and pharmacology at Duke. Shortly thereafter he went to the University of Chicago to become the dean of their medical school, and he preempted me by submitting a smaller grant to the Commonwealth Fund for the same purpose. I don't know how it fared at Chicago, but we did get our grant, and it had lasting impact (though some of the trustees of the Commonwealth Fund probably felt that it was a waste of their money).

When the grant ended, collaborative endeavors between the Medical Center and the university's Schools of Arts and Sciences and Engineering continued to flourish. There are now strong and developing academic bonds between them. A recently developed program is one in genomic sciences, which brings together many components of the university to look at the legal and ethical components of advances in genetics. The Divinity School has always had a major joint program in hospital chaplaincy; recently it has developed a joint program with the School of Nursing in parish nursing. An outstanding, unifying program is housed in the new Levine Research Building, where components of the biological sciences are housed with collaborative units of the engineering, computer, and medical sciences. What started as collaborative programs scattered across the campus such as molecular biology, genetics, and biomedical engineering are now housed under one roof to enhance their activities.

I think physicians should be very roundly educated individuals, interested in a lifetime of education, which includes reading a number of publications such as the *New York Times*, many magazines, and books that have nothing to do with medicine. I was particularly fortunate to have attended an English school and consequently to have received an extensive liberal arts education. I don't think that kind of education is readily available in the United States. Nonetheless, in selecting the students coming into medicine, we should assess how well the individual is educated in subjects other than science and include in our assessment such free-time activities as reading and writing, as well as traditional hobbies.

A physician should be able to relate to patients on a human—not just a scientific—level, although I do not think that an undergraduate liberal arts education guarantees that skill. I remember one year we had an applicant from Davidson College, an excellent liberal arts institution. A Duke trustee from the Charlotte area told me that we had turned down this young man, even though he was number 2 in his class at Davidson, with a 4.2 average. My first question was, "How do you get a 4.2 out of 4?" I learned that if you do extracurricular work at Davidson, they give you a bonus. So I called Syd Osterhout, who was dean of admissions at the Medical School, and asked him why we didn't accept this young man. His response was one I shall never forget: "Well, this young man has done nothing but study all day long. The only time he leaves his room is to hit a tennis ball against the wall, playing alone. He has no socializing skills. How would you like him to walk into your hospital room when you are sick?" He made his point. I have the utmost respect for the screening that the Medical School's admissions committee gives to the thousands of applicants a year who compete for the school's one hundred slots.

As far as continuing medical education—designed to keep practicing physicians current in particular fields—is concerned, we probably know better what not to do than what really works. As it has turned out, there are countless ways of staying current in your field, from reading and using computers and the Internet to attending national meetings such as those sponsored by the American College of Surgery or American College of Physicians, which offer specific courses in a variety of fields. Physicians today, to maintain their licensures in states such as North Carolina, must register the number of hours they have attended lectures or seminars, although that does not mean that they were present intellectually as well as physically.

You can be asleep during those lectures and conferences and still chalk up the time. I think the system is far too lenient and permissive in this respect. The situation is worse in England, where the general practitioner is paid a significant bonus for attending continuing education courses, all of which start out with cocktails and a three-course lunch followed by two-and-a-half hours or so of lectures, when many members of the audience are fast asleep.

Some medical schools have large continuing medical education programs, others have small, quality programs, which I think is more the case with Duke. We also have to remember that these programs bear some relationship to patient referrals, especially for primary care physicians, in that the specialists who teach in these programs tend to get referrals from generalists who have heard them talk about a given problem.

There is one area where I feel that I failed, and that is with the Program in Hospital Administration, or health administration as it is now called. It was probably the earliest educational program in the Medical Center. Dr. Davison and the first superintendent of the Duke hospital, M. E. Winston, thought it was important to train hospital administrators. The program was based on the idea that teaching hospitals should seek out "keen" university graduates who had specialized in economics and sociology, and train them as hospital administrators and future hospital superintendents. When I came to Duke in 1949, the program was mainly a tutorial experience, with rotations of the students in various administrative offices both at Duke and elsewhere, including the administrative offices of The Duke Endowment in Charlotte, where the hospital section was housed. The first two interns—F. Vernon Altvater and F. Ross Porter—in due time became the Duke hospital's superintendent and assistant superintendent, respectively. When Ross Porter retired, Charles Frenzel, a product of the program, was his successor as superintendent of Duke Hospital. (Subsequently the title was changed to "director of Duke Hospital.")

Charlie Frenzel succeeded in getting the graduate school of Duke University to formalize health administration as a master's degree program. The idea was a promising one, and it is to his credit that it got off the ground. Frenzel and the people involved in the program recruited Ray Brown, who had been director of the University of Chicago Hospitals and Clinics and other national programs, to come to Duke in 1964 to head the new program. Brown was a delightful person, but he did not spend much time in Durham because he was very much in demand for lectures around the country. He left after a couple of years, going to Harvard to head their affiliated hospitals (with the exception of Massachusetts General). We had a series of people visit as potential successors of Ray Brown, with Charlie Frenzel holding the fort when we were looking for a new leader. Unfortunately, after Ray Brown's departure the program never achieved the quality to match the Medical School.

When the Fuqua School of Business was developed at Duke, Tom Keller, as the first significant head of that school, offered to take over the program as part of the business school. I felt that Tom's main interest was to reach into the pockets of the hospital section of The Duke Endowment, and therefore I resisted until 1989, when I left the Medical Center.

A series of leaders of the program never quite succeeded in making it a program of good quality. In fact, in the mid-1980s, the university decided that the first-year students would take their core courses with the first-year students at Fuqua, and it further decided that the Health Administration Program should be limited to around 30 students each year. Even so, a sufficient number of students continued to apply for admission each year.

After Alex McMahon retired as president of the American Hospital Association in 1986, I prevailed on him to come and spearhead the Program in Health Administration since he was exceptionally qualified and anxious to get back to the Duke-Durham scene. He did this very successfully for a number of years, but it was decided in the early 1990s, for a number of reasons, that the future of the Health Administration Program would be better served if it were moved in its entirety to the Fuqua School of Business, a move that occurred in the summer of 1992. In the early years at Fuqua, the program lost students, averaging around 15 instead of the 30 or so it had in its last years in the Medical Center. It has, however, since grown: in the 2002–2003 academic year there were 54 health center management students enrolled in Fuqua's first-year class of 350 day students and 52 health sector management students in the second-year class, and the program receives strong support from the Fuqua administration.

8

RAISING THE MONEY

ONE OF MY FUNCTIONS in leading the Medical Center was to provide the means to finance its growth and development. This was known as fund-raising. I had some limited experience raising money for my own laboratory projects from both the NIH and the American Cancer Society, but this was not fund-raising on the scale demanded from the head of the Medical Center.

The first major grant that I solicited and that we were fortunate to get shortly after I became dean was from the Commonwealth Fund of New York, to help implement the Medical School's new curriculum. That was the first time I recall going after big private money.

I have found that many of the people who have large amounts of money for private philanthropy either never went to college or did not finish the usual four years. Examples include Jack Whitehead, J. B. Fuqua, and Dave Thomas. Others who did go to college were very individualistic and had to be cultivated for quite some time. It was helpful if they or their families had been patients at Duke. The one thing that I always tried to impress on the small staff I had in development—which is what fund-raising is rather euphemistically called in academic institutions, and which started in the Medical Center with one person and then built up to a handful—was to insist that they not rush, but that they devote a certain amount of time to cultivating individuals. After all, it took President Few twelve years to convince James B. Duke to make his magnificent gift to create Duke University.

The Medical Center is big business today—and has been, almost from its start. I would guess that the Medical Center budget accounts for about 60 to 65 percent of the total Duke University budget and that about 60 percent of the faculty is in the Medical Center. (Contrast this with the situation at Yale, where the medical center accounts for about 45 to 50 percent of the total budget, because the Yale–New Haven Hospital is a separate corporate entity. Once you put a teaching hospital into the equation, as we do at Duke, the figures change dramatically.)

In the course of raising money to support this large enterprise, I met many wonderful people and some challenging ones. One of the more memorable was Doris Duke. Doris Duke was one of the richest women in the world. More to the point in the context of my work, she was the daughter of James B. Duke, the man who had founded Duke University and established The Duke Endowment. While her word may not have been law at Duke, it certainly carried heavy, heavy weight, as I was to discover in the late sixties.

Doris Duke had made the acquaintance of one Kenneth S. MacLean in New York. Dr. MacLean was a Canadian with an M.D. from McGill Medical School, who trained as an obstetrician-gynecologist at Royal Victoria Hospital in Montreal and at Doctors Hospital and Roosevelt Hospital in New York. He headed an institute of biomagnetics, where he used magnetic force to treat a variety of ills, ranging all the way from lack of energy to cancer and heart disease. Doris Duke's principal interest in MacLean was that he treated her for chronic fatigue, that he literally "recharged her batteries" by having her lie in a magnetic field. Miss Duke felt that MacLean's treatment also had rejuvenating effects, so she had become not only a patient but also a disciple of his. Periodically, Dr. MacLean would pack his batteries and magnet and charter a plane to fly out to treat Doris wherever she was at the time, be it California or Honolulu, Thailand or Paris.

Although MacLean had accumulated a dossier of letters from doctors who testified to the efficacy of his treatments, his method had not been received with open arms by the medical community. No reputable—or for that matter, disreputable—medical center had run any tests to substantiate his claims.

The MacLean matter came up at Duke University Medical Center when Dr. Davison was contacted by MacLean. Miss Duke had requested that Duke run some trials of MacLean's methods. Davison thereupon contacted Bob Gregg, professor of physical medicine and rehabilitation, who had received a small grant from Doris Duke's foundation. At some point, Dr. Gregg thought that he was in over his head, and he asked for my help.

From the correspondence over this episode (eventually, I had to prepare what amounted to a legal brief on the whole matter), I have been able to reconstruct how it unfolded. I went to see Dr. Davison, who was very supportive of Dr. MacLean. I felt, however, that very little was known about the effect of magnetic fields on biological systems, and the closest people to the field at Duke were the radiobiologists in the Department of Radiology. As was my usual approach, I went through the chairman, at that time Dick Lester, whom I had just recruited to Duke, and he contacted Aaron Sanders, who was a radiobiologist and a radio-isotope man and thus probably came closest of anyone at Duke to working with magnetic fields.

Both Dr. Sanders and Dr. Lester visited Dr. MacLean. We caucused after they came back and felt that we could not dismiss the matter out of hand, so we agreed to set up an experimental lab, hoping it would be partially supported by Doris Duke, to study the effect of magnetic fields on living biological systems. I remember in one conversation with Doris, when I told her we were willing to do this, she said, "You are not going to use dogs and cats, are you?" I said, "No, this will be done on mice and rats," and she said, "Thank goodness." She was a very strong animal lover and a champion of animal rights.

Somewhere along the line I decided it was time for me to visit Mac-Lean and, separately, to visit Doris Duke. MacLean was in a dingy third-floor walk-up in a townhouse in mid-town Manhattan. In the middle of a large room stood a huge magnet, probably several feet across and from top to bottom, mounted vertically and powered by six automobile batteries because the health department of Manhattan had turned off the power source to the magnet. MacLean came across to me not as a quack but more as a schizophrenic individual, who seemed out of touch with reality and very nervous about what he was trying to tell me. He had a lot of slides of patients before their treatment, but none of the same patients after treatment. In order to show me what he did, he had me hold a large hammer with a steel head in between the poles of the magnet. Then he threw a big switch to activate the power from the automobile batteries and just about wrenched my shoulder out of joint as one of the magnetic poles attracted the hammer. There was, indeed, a magnetic field.

Subsequently, when I visited Doris, we had a lovely tea in her Manhattan apartment overlooking Central Park. I explained to her that so little was known of the effect of magnetic fields on biological systems that we proposed doing this research project for a modest amount of money. Everything seemed to be just fine when I left. As a matter of fact, one of the buttons fell off my jacket onto her shaggy rug, and she was kind enough to take off her shoes and walk around barefoot trying to find my button (without success). As I left New York to fly to a meeting in Washington, I kept wondering why people felt that she was a difficult woman. She was very charming, very friendly, and seemed to understand what I was proposing.

Not too long after that she called me from Honolulu, and her tone of voice was ice cold. She said that she understood that I wasn't going to use this machine on humans. She was very, very angry, and at one point she hung up. I assume this was the point at which she activated her channels to Dr. Davison, who became very rude to me in subsequent phone calls, telling me such things as, "What the hell difference does it make if you move the damn machine to Durham and just put some patients under it and satisfy Doris?" I explained to Dr. Davison that this was unethical and bordered on the immoral, and that the institution he built and that I was trying to develop further would be jeopardized for treating patients with an unproven therapy. It certainly was against any of the guidelines of the U.S. surgeon general in terms of acceptable new treatments. Dr. Davison went so far as to call me up one evening when I was in Minneapolis having dinner with Lewis Wannamaker, who was a candidate for the chair in pediatrics. Dr. Davison insisted I be called to the phone, whereupon he became quite rude. It was the only time I ever hung up on anybody.

It was not too long after that that I learned that Dr. Davison had asked the executive committee of the university trustees to have me fired as the dean by Duke University President Knight. When Doug Knight got the word, he asked me to fly back from a Markle scholar meeting at Hot Springs, Virginia, to appear before the executive committee and to present my case. When I finished making my presentation to the executive committee, Tom Perkins, who was also chairman of the board of The Duke Endowment and a former lawyer of Doris Duke's, and who had also at some point disagreed with her, made the motion to the committee to clear my name and to support what I had done. He was seconded by Marshall Pickens, who, in addition to being on the executive committee of the Duke University trustees, was also vice chairman of The Duke Endowment Board of Trustees. The vote was unanimous in support of what I had done. After that, I never heard another negative word from Davison, and in his last few years we got along fine.

Another major donor was Disque Deane. We first met in the early seventies. Deane had made his money as a senior managing partner of Lazard Frères; he had also been in the real estate business around New York as well as in other parts of the hemisphere. John Thomas, of my fund-raising staff, had identified him as a potential donor. Deane at that time was living in a midtown Manhattan townhouse. He was a Duke alumnus but had not been connected to Duke in any way since his graduation.

He agreed to give a small dinner party in my honor, and John Thomas and I were to arrive at his house around 6:30 P.M. That particular day was an especially hectic one because I had just finished working on details of a possible Whitehead Institute at Duke University with Jack Whitehead and his consultant, Jim Shannon, the former NIH director. We got to the airport, only to find that Eastern Airlines had canceled our flight; the best we could do was take a United Airlines flight that landed in Newark considerably later than the appointed hour. We alerted Disque that there would be a delay in our arrival, that we did not know the magnitude of that delay, but that we would keep him informed. Unfortunately, he did not hang up the phone, so when we tried to reach him in the ensuing hours, the line was busy.

When we finally boarded the United Airlines flight, we realized that Dr. Shannon had been helping himself liberally to the alcoholic refreshments in the Eastern Airlines lounge. He continued to ask for refreshments while on board. We got to Newark about 8 P.M. and found a cab willing to drive us to Manhattan. When I noticed the cabdriver taking the Pulaski Skyway instead of the Lincoln Tunnel, I asked him why he was doing that; he said he was a Cuban refugee and had never actually driven this taxi into New York. We managed to get to Jim Shannon's apartment, which was near the Deanes' house, and get him into it, then dropped off Jack Whitehead, and proceeded immediately to the Deane home.

By the time we got there, around 9:15, Disque Deane had become annoyed at not hearing from us. He had been wearing evening clothes, but he was already in his bedroom changing into his nightclothes. His wife was sitting alone at the head of the table. The help who were to serve the meal were upset because they had opened the wines at just the right time to be served, and the dinner itself was partially burned. The saving grace was that when we explained that the phone must be off the hook, Deane checked, and indeed it was. So we stumbled through the rest of the evening. I was never so glad to get into a hotel and into bed. Shortly afterward, Terry Sanford appointed Disque Deane to the Duke University Board of Trustees, and he would come to meetings once in a while.

Disque came to the groundbreaking ceremony and the luncheon for the Bryan Research Building for Neurobiology, having been invited along with the other trustees. That afternoon, he appeared in my office and said he would like to talk to me the next time I was in New York because of his intense interest in neurobiology. At some point he had been or was a trustee of Rockefeller University, which no doubt fed this interest.

I made sure that I would be in New York within a couple of weeks. He consented to see me, but when I appeared in his office, he apologized that he had forgotten that this was the day he was hosting his annual office Christmas party at the floating restaurant on the East River, and asked if I would mind going with him. Three hours later, after a massive luncheon and dancing with all the secretaries, I thanked him and left it that we would schedule another visit to get down to the business of neurobiology.

After the first of that year, Duke President Terry Sanford and his major fund-raiser, Joel Fleishman, decided to initiate an endowment campaign for professorships in the arts and sciences. I was informed that Disque Deane would no longer be on my list of potential donors, but that he would be assigned to Joel Fleishman. In the ensuing many months, Joel spent a lot of time cultivating Mr. Deane for a series of professorships in the Institute for Public Policy. Mr. Deane never quite understood what the main thrust of the program was to be, and he was frustrated because his primary interest continued to be in neurobiology. Finally, Joel arranged for a substantial press conference and an announcement of a $20 million pledge from Mr. Deane—who told me later he did not know what he was signing when he was rushed into putting his name on a document. From then on, he was extremely hostile to and angry with the Duke Campaign for the Arts and Sciences.

The university's announcement had included the statement that the $20 million pledge would make Mr. Deane the biggest single contributor to Duke University in the private field. This alienated Joseph Bryan, who felt that, next to James Buchanan Duke, he had been the largest contributor to various causes at Duke. So I had to put out the fire with Mr. Bryan and mend that fence. Subsequently, after Disque Deane had been written off by the university, I was handed back his folder.

For a few years I visited Mr. Deane on a regular basis when I was in New York. At times he would get very angry with me, because I was a symbol of Duke University, and he would recite all the problems he had had with the staff of the university campaign. At some point I put him in touch with Allen Roses, chief of neurology, and they developed a good relationship. Mr. Deane initially gave us three $1.5 million professorships. Beyond that,

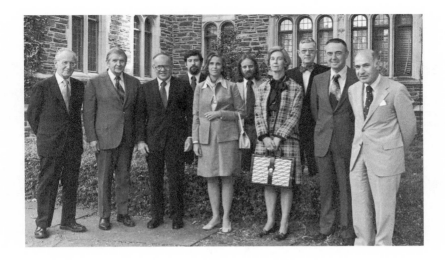

12   The Whitehead Institute Advisory Board on the occasion of their site visit in 1972 to consider Duke as the site of the institute. (Front row, L–R): Dr. Irving Page, Cleveland Clinic; President Terry Sanford, Duke University; Jack and Betsy Whitehead; Mr. Whitehead's assistant; Dr. Leonard Skeggs; (back row, L–R): Arthur Brill, legal counsel for Mr. Whitehead; John Whitehead, son of Mr. Whitehead; Dr. James Shannon, former director of the National Institutes of Health. DUMC Photography.

he established the Deane Laboratories in Neurobiology in the Department of Medicine for another $6–7 million.

Edwin C. (Jack) Whitehead was another challenge. In 1939 he and his father had founded Technicon, a maker of scientific and laboratory equipment. In 1972 he had sold Technicon and ended up with about $120 million from the sale with which he wanted to establish a biomedical research institute. He brought together a very distinguished panel of scientists to advise him on allying his institute with a suitable academic institution, and at the completion of the first round, competing with all the topnotch universities, Duke was chosen as the home for the nascent Whitehead Institute. In subsequent negotiations, however, it became clear that Mr. Whitehead wanted not only to be on the board of the Whitehead Institute as well as on the Board of Trustees of Duke University but also to be able to nominate 51 percent or more of the board of the institute, thus controlling all of the appointments. It was on this matter that he and I parted ways, or we reached "a Mexican standoff," as he called it, and he decided that Duke was not the place where he wanted to put the institute. But I was not willing to sell quality control over faculty and scientists of the university to satisfy the whims of Mr. Whitehead. Throughout this whole period his son, John Whitehead, was never quite comfortable with the Duke decision and had been very eager to place the institute in Boston, preferably at MIT, where it ended up.

In the course of parting with Jack Whitehead (we remained close friends in spite of the preceding), he called me up one day and wanted to give a $1 million consolation prize to Duke University Medical Center. I was at my home at Beech Mountain at the time, and I was about to pick up the phone to call him directly, but instead I wrote him a nasty letter, telling him what I thought he ought to do with the million dollars. Fortuitously, the letter never got to him because the person who was to carry it back to Durham to have it transcribed forgot to take it. Overnight I decided that one catches more flies with honey than with anything else, so instead of a nasty letter, I wrote him a glowing letter of praise and said that the minimum price for parting would be $10 million. About three weeks later he called me up, and his words were, "Dammit, Bill, you're right. I'm going to make $10 million available to Duke." After his death, his three children and the Whitehead Foundation have gone well beyond the $10 million in their support of the Medical Center. His daughter, Susan Whitehead, is chair of the board of the Whitehead Biomedical Research Institute at MIT, and she invited me to serve on their board of advisors. She is a talented lawyer who has also served on some Duke University advisory boards.

In addition, Jack founded Research!America, a group that is the private-sector advocate for increased funding for biomedical research, and he invited me to serve on the board. A few years later, when he died unexpectedly on the tennis court at his home in Greenwich, the trustees asked me to succeed him as chairman of the board, which I did for four years, laying the groundwork for what Research!America is today. (I was fortunate to have former U.S. representative Paul Rogers, a partner of Hogan & Hartson in Washington, succeed me. Paul has done an outstanding job. It has also been a pleasure serving on the board of Research!America with John Whitehead, who has become a pillar of the organization.)

Another interesting fund-raising episode concerned Ray Nasher and Duke's art museum. Ray had been identified as a potential major donor by the university's alumni office, and he had indicated early in his career that he had an interest in the Medical School and the Medical Center. Therefore, as we were forming the Medical Center's Board of Visitors in the mid-sixties, we invited him to join us. Ray had a very successful track record building shopping centers in Florida and Texas as a real estate developer. He was very helpful as we looked at capital improvements in the Medical Center expansion. As a result of his success on the Duke University Medical Center Board of Visitors, he was invited to join the Duke University Board of Trustees.

I got to know Ray Nasher and his wife, Patsy, reasonably well, and we enjoyed playing tennis on the court at their home in Dallas. They were very proud of their art collection, which included a substantial number of important works of outdoor sculpture, notably Henry Moore. Subsequently, when Mike Mezzatesta came from Fort Worth to head up the art museum at Duke, he was thoroughly familiar with Ray Nasher and, as a result, Ray became a prime figure in Duke's planning for a new art museum. Up to then, Duke's art collection had been housed in a fairly obscure part of the campus. To continue to build Duke's collection, it was considered vital to put the museum into more fitting and more accessible quarters.

Nasher's preferred piece of land on the Duke campus conflicted with the experimental work of a botany professor who had been studying a group of unusual weeds on the property, and Ray got very upset—and so did his family, including his daughter Nancy, a Duke law graduate who has since become a Duke trustee—and thus any conversations about the museum were discontinued. The figure that had been dangled in front of Mr. Nasher was $3 million. When I became chancellor of the university in 1989, Keith Brodie, as university president, asked me to mend the fences with Ray Nasher. It took several visits and coordination with Mike Mezzatesta, but subsequently we got on a positive track again. In the meantime, the price tag had escalated to $6–7 million, but the botany professor and his graduate students have completed their project on the property Nasher wanted and recently he confirmed the gift that will be coming to the new art museum.

Ed Benenson, too, supported both the university and the Medical Center. He had attended Duke for three years, and in recent years has had the courage and perseverance to complete his undergraduate degree as a senior citizen. He is well known in the worlds of real estate, art, and wine. He has made numerous contributions to components of the university, including the art museum, and to the Medical Center, supporting several scholarships and fellowships. He was also very effective on the Medical Center's board of visitors, and subsequently he became a member not only of the full Duke

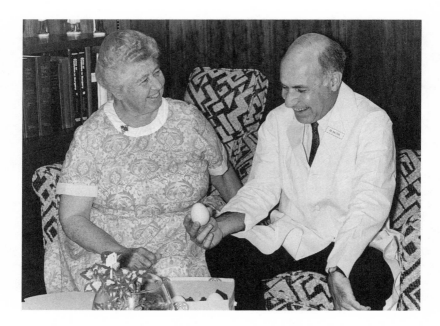

13   Dr. W. G. Anlyan with Miss Betty Dumaine, a major supporter of programs of
the Medical Center, who introduced key national and international people to the
campus, including Queen Sirikit of Thailand. DUMC Photography.

University Board of Trustees but also of its executive committee. For many
years, Ed and his wife, Gladys, have hosted a luncheon at the Palm Beach
Country Club, hosting speakers and the leadership of the Medical Center
each March.

Betty Dumaine, the daughter of a New England textile tycoon, was identified by John Thomas as a person I should get to know. I invited her to
Duke as a member of various visiting boards. In turn, she appointed me
to her board of the Princess Mother's Foundation. The Princess Mother
was the mother of the King of Thailand. She had been Betty Dumaine's
roommate in prep school and now had a foundation based in the United
States, with Betty Dumaine as its head. The foundation supported a variety
of small health programs in Thailand, especially the northern rural part of
the country. All the other board members were old friends of Betty Dumaine's; most of them had either served in the armed forces in Southeast
Asia, like General Joseph Stilwell, or had been in the CIA at one time or
another around Thailand. It was an informal, closely knit group that met

approximately twice a year for dinner at Betty Dumaine's home in Pinehurst, N.C. John Thomas, who was quite a good friend of Miss Dumaine's,
always accompanied me on those trips. I remember the first night I spent
at her house, after one of the board meetings. I was awakened in the middle
of the night by a series of bloodcurdling screams. I did not know that she
raised peacocks and thought someone was being put away in the backyard.

Elliott Richardson and I were "adopted nephews" of Betty Dumaine's.
Richardson may have had a blood connection, but certainly there was none
between Betty and me. In her will, she left all portable materials in her Pinehurst estate to Richardson and all the fixed furnishings to me and in turn to
Duke University; I had no personal gain in this bequest. When Betty Dumaine died, John Thomas and I went to her memorial service and before
her ashes were sprinkled around her favorite riding area, Elliott Richardson
gave a very touching and emotional eulogy. In fact, he could hardly finish
his comments. At the end of her life, Betty weighed about 350 pounds, and
it is hard to visualize her bouncing around on a horse in a hunt in Pinehurst.

John Thomas was one of my more important associates in fund-raising
because he had a knack for dealing with wealthy but difficult people. He
was particularly good at spending the appropriate amount of time with
widows, and seeing that their needs were met when they came to Duke for
medical treatment. John did not fit the mold of the typical fund-raising person; when I tried to fit him into the development group that R. C. (Bucky)
Waters (the former Duke basketball coach, now on my staff) was putting
together, it did not work. Therefore, I had John as a "soloist" reporting directly to me, without being part of the evolving development office. When
I later became chancellor of the university, I took John and Janet Sanfilippo,
another senior staff assistant, with me, and John continued to be helpful
in a variety of ways. After I resigned as chancellor and went to The Duke
Endowment, I tried to place John in the university or Medical Center development office, but as he was not the kind of person the people in charge
were looking for, he was, unfortunately, left without a job.

Nancy "Trink" Gardiner was one of the more remarkable friends of the
Medical Center during my era. An heiress to the John Deere tractor fortune, she had at one time been married to William Wakeman, who had
become a paraplegic when she shot him in 1967. (She was convicted of
aggravated assault and sentenced to five years probation; this conviction
was reversed on appeal.) After Mr. Wakeman's death, Trink married Win-
throp J. Gardiner. Their divorce also made headlines, because he was one of
the first men to ask for substantial alimony from a wealthy wife. Each year

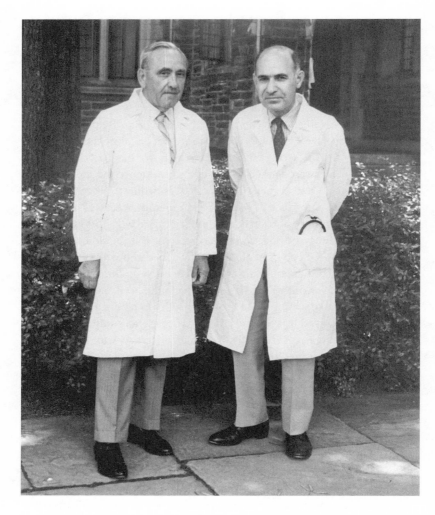

14 Mr. Henry M. Rauch, former chairman of the board of Burlington Industries and vice chairman of the Duke University Board of Trustees, later chairman of the Medical Center's Board of Visitors and a key supporter in the planning of Duke Hospital North. DUMC Photography.

Mrs. Gardiner would host a cocktail party and dinner at her home, inviting all our alumni and friends in the Palm Beach area. Many of those friends came to Duke for their medical care.

In subsequent years Mrs. Gardiner befriended a number of other paraplegics, and in 1972 she established the Wakeman Award for scientists doing the best work in spinal cord regeneration research. With the help of Jim and Mary Semans, we persuaded Mrs. Gardiner to have Duke University Medical Center operate the award, much as the Nobel Prizes in biomedicine are administered by the Karolinska Institute in Sweden. Jim Semans, a urologist, was long interested in spinal cord injuries because of the effect they have on the urogenital tract, and he was very well connected on the national scene with organizations interested in paraplegia. I persuaded Allen Roses, as head of the division of neurology, to take the lead in setting up this biannual award, which has been a very successful venture. Some of the recipients of the Wakeman Award have gone on to win the Nobel Prize in medicine. In 1986 Mrs. Gardiner established a $1 million endowment for the Wakeman Award for Research in the Neurosciences. The award did a very effective job of bringing spinal cord research to the public eye in the years before Christopher Reeves's accident brought an even higher focus on this tragic problem. Mrs. Gardiner died in 1996.

Not all major gifts can be measured in dollars; sometimes the gift is expertise and time. Three key figures supporting me in the seventies, as we approached a decision on the construction of the new hospital, contributed immeasurably in nonmonetary ways: Alex McMahon, Terry Sanford, and Henry Rauch.

I was very fortunate in having Alex McMahon as chairman of the Duke University Board of Trustees and a member of the Medical Center's Board of Visitors at that time. Alex had been running N.C. Blue Cross and Blue Shield, and in the early seventies he was made president of the American Hospital Association. He was thoroughly conversant with all our problems and needs at the Medical Center. Alex and I developed a firm and long-standing personal friendship. As a matter of fact, in 1976 we set about planning the Private Sector Conferences as a way of bringing together the major associations in the field of medicine and health care in the nation. When Alex retired in the late eighties, he came back to live in the Durham area, and I persuaded him to head up our floundering Health Administration Program, which he did very effectively, capping off his many contributions to the university, in general, and to the Medical Center, in particular.

The second person who helped the Medical Center immeasurably during my time there was Duke University President, Terry Sanford, who was very comfortable making major decisions and handling big money. Many of the things that were accomplished in my time were thanks to the unfailing support of President Sanford. He and I developed a special relationship of mutual respect.

Henry Rauch, the vice chairman of Duke University's board of trustees, had been chairman of the board of Burlington Industries. He was a very astute businessman with a background in accounting, and his judgment was greatly respected by the other trustees. If Henry said it was okay financially, they could rest at ease. Because of his position on the board of trustees, I invited him in the mid-sixties to become chairman of the Board of Visitors, which he did. He soon was so much on top of everything that went on at the Medical Center that he kept at least three of my staff busy working figures till the budgets met with his satisfaction. In 1972, when it came down to the votes by the Duke University Board of Trustees for the go-ahead on planning and constructing the new hospital, Mr. Rauch told the board that he insisted that we have sure pledges for 40 percent of the anticipated $95 million expenditure. He carried the day, and of course we met his minimum requirement. With Mr. Rauch's help we recruited John Shytle, previously a major figure in the Veterans Administration, who for many years did an outstanding job as financial officer of the Medical Center as we built and operated the new hospital. In sum, Mr. Rauch was enormously helpful. He contributed in large measure by the leadership that he exercised.

Fund-raising is a two-edged sword. Obviously, a private institution such as Duke's Medical Center depends heavily on outside funding, from both public sources — like the NIH — and private sources — donors large and small. Some people in this institution consider fund-raising an impediment to their "real" work. Some people like the contact with a great many people, not to mention the challenge fund-raising undoubtedly presents. Successful fund-raising really depends on the person and his or her personality. President Terry Sanford was audacious in asking people who did not expect to be asked for amounts that were far in excess of anything they had remotely had in mind.

I think I was closer to Terry Sanford's style and I enjoyed it, provided I knew what I was getting into. I always made sure that the homework had been done — that I knew the person's background, attitude, and connections toward Duke, and had some idea of the financial capabilities — and that what I was requesting was something of interest to the person I was

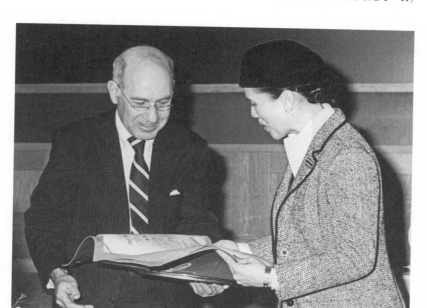

15 Queen Sirikit of Thailand exchanging books with Dr. W. G. Anlyan on the occasion of her visit to Duke, February 18, 1980. DUMC Photography.

meeting and the figure was not outlandish. When I asked the Searle family for $1 million to create the Searle Center out of the shell space that was in the Seeley G. Mudd Building, it was almost a shot in the dark. On the other hand, when John Thomas, of our fund-raising team, and I had breakfast with Roger Milliken, the longtime CEO of Milliken mills in South Carolina, and I asked him for $5 million or $10 million, which we knew he could very easily have afforded, he practically went into shock and we never heard from him again. In the middle ground is someone like Leon Levine, whom I approached for a gift of $25 million, then was happy to settle for $10 million toward the Levine Science Research Center. You have to be flexible and willing to accept either a totally negative response, a nonresponse, or something in between.

Dr. Barth Geller was a successful practicing physician in New York City who retired in 1946 and moved to Fort Lauderdale, Florida. He was interested in leaving his estate to medical research. He was originally interested in the Damon Runyan Fund for Cancer Research. In discussing possibilities with his attorney, John Douglas in Fort Lauderdale, the question of considering the Duke Medical Center was raised. I was invited to visit Dr. Geller. Mr. Douglas arranged for a luncheon in Fort Lauderdale. Dr. Geller was a widower and despite his age, which I guessed to be in the mid-eighties, he was very lucid and specific about his interests in cancer and heart disease. I had no idea about the size of his estate. My guess was a few million because of the growth of his investments combined with a spartan lifestyle. Thereafter for many years, John Douglas and I would visit him once a year. After 1989 I invited Ralph Snyderman to accompany us; we would schedule our visits around the time of the Benenson luncheon in Palm Beach. When Dr. Geller died in his mid-nineties, his estate amounted to $16 million and was earmarked to support several professorships at Duke in the fields of cancer, cardiovascular research, immunology, genetics, neurobiology, molecular biology, and pharmacology. These professorships have been key to attracting and retaining distinguished faculty at the Medical Center. The whole story is exemplary of what I have often thought, that cultivating lawyers is an important part of development work. In this instance, John Douglas's interest was related to the fact that his brother, Fenner Douglas, was the university organist. In the negotiations with John, the question of possible support of the organist was raised; however, when Fenner left the university, we settled on having one of the professorships in chemistry.

The Davison Club deserves special mention in the annals of our Medical Center fund-raising. It is the $1,000-a-year club of Medical Center supporters—mainly alumnae and alumni, but also grateful patients and people who simply want to support medical excellence. It has been invaluable in many, many ways, and it came about out of pure necessity.

When I became dean in 1964, there were no discretionary funds in the dean's office. The dean's salary was $25,000 a year. There was only an endowment of $2.7 million from the initial Ford grant that it had received many years before. There was just one scholarship, and it was for $500 for a "white Methodist," preferably male, from Charlotte, and it covered the entire four years of medical school. So we set about looking for discretionary moneys—that is, funds that could be used as needs arose and for funding for scholarships.

About that time, Dr. Joe Hiatt came to see me and told me that Chapel Hill was starting a $1,000-a-year club and that we ought to consider doing the same thing. Joe was a Duke alumnus practicing in Pinehurst in internal medicine. His very close friend and colleague, Bill Hollister, was a distinguished surgeon, trained at Duke, in the same community. Shortly after the idea was planted, there was a meeting of seven of us in Dr. Jay Arena's study: Joe Hiatt, Jay Arena, John Robert Kernodle, Bill Hollister, John Yarborough, Dr. Davison himself, and me. All were Duke medical alumni. Over a little bourbon, we persuaded Davison that it would be a good thing to start this $1,000-a-year club in his name. Of course, $1,000 in the sixties was a lot of money, though not out of line with what many of our alumni could afford, and finally Dr. Davison agreed to lend his name to the club, which has become an outstanding success—not only in raising much-needed funds but in creating a strong family of Duke supporters.

Soon after the Davison Club had its first formal meeting in 1969, it became apparent that we needed a person full-time to help recruit members and run the club. The first person to take up the post was Charlie Smith— the Reverend Charles Smith—then a recent graduate of the Duke Divinity School. I felt that at least he would know how to pray for money, but actually he knew a lot more than that, because he did very well, and after leaving our post he continued to climb the ladder in his field. He is now a trustee of Duke University. The second person I recruited was Gerry Hancock, then a recent graduate of Duke Law School. Gerry had had an accident before working with me, and he had only one eye. Driving around with someone you know has only one eye can be somewhat harrowing—but Gerry did extremely well. After leaving us, he became a state senator and has had a thriving law career. Just about then, Bucky Waters was looking around for something bigger and better to do than coach basketball teams. We were delighted to recruit him to head our alumni and Davison Club programs. He has also done very well as a sports commentator on TV while fulfilling his responsibilities at Duke Medical Center as vice chancellor for development.

The Davison Club has, I think, done the best job of all in providing a solid financial basis for a great many of our efforts with fluid funds—and in helping in yet another way to cement our relationship with our ever expanding family of friends and alumni. By 1999 we had about seven hundred paying members, who that year alone contributed $1.4 million to Duke's medical enterprise. Over the first thirty years of its existence, the club had contributed a total of $13 million.

At this point, it might be pertinent to quote Dr. Davison: "A medical school is only as good as its alumni. After all, they are its major product, and by their fruits, ye shall know them." In some institutions, alumni loyalty is based upon the place and building. In others, on the faculty, or on the football team, or on fraternities. But the alumni loyalty built upon the close friendships of a well-organized class, as at Duke, not only provides Duke with active alumni support but also gives each member of the class the opportunity of cementing in after-years the close ties which had developed in college. Keeping these friendships alive by frequent reunions, class dinners and luncheons, and news notes about each other not only adds to the pleasure of the members of the class, but frequently is a source of mutual help. In this, as in so many other instances, "the dean" had it right.

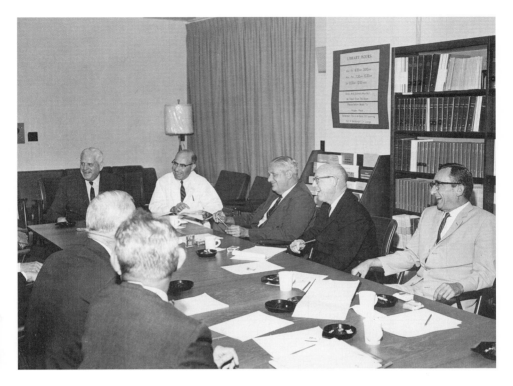

1   The three medical school deans of North Carolina, Dr. William G. Anlyan of Duke, Dr. Manson
Meads of the Bowman Gray School of Medicine, and Dr. Isaac Taylor of the UNC School of Medi-
cine, meeting with the leadership of the N.C. Medical Society to discuss the establishment of the
N.C. Regional Medical Programs for Heart, Cancer and Stroke; Dr. George Paschal, president of
N.C. Medical Society, presiding. 1965. DUMC Photography.

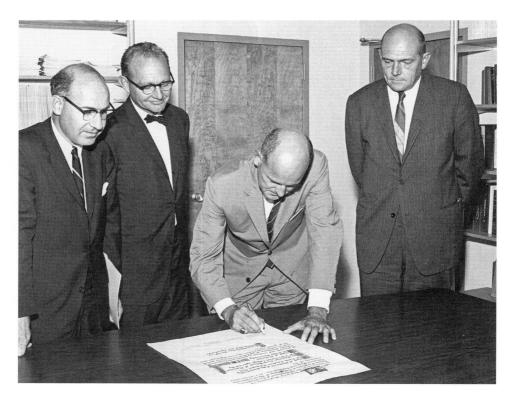

2 The first joint endeavor of the three medical school deans of North Carolina: signing an agreement to run a new biomedical research laboratory in Wrightsville Beach. (L–R): Dr. W. G. Anlyan; Dr. Manson Meads; Mr. Wright, chairman of the board of the laboratory; and Dr. Isaac Taylor. 1965. DUMC Photography.

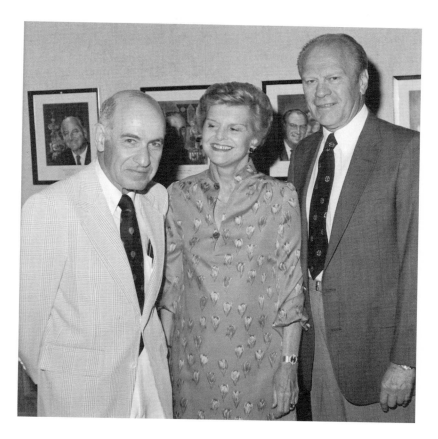

3 Former President and Mrs. Ford on the occasion of their participation in the 1982 Duke Children's Classic, a major fund-raising event for Duke Children's Hospital. DUMC Photography.

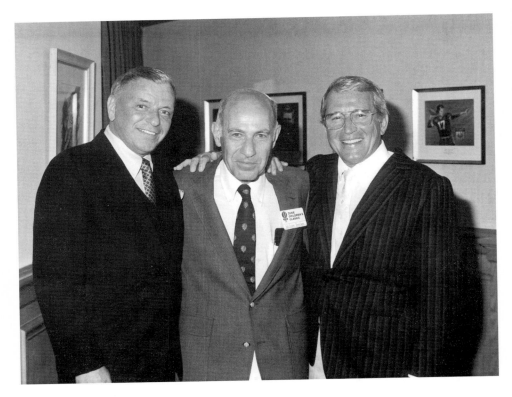

4   Frank Sinatra and Perry Como just before their performance at the Celebrity Program of the 1982 Duke Children's Classic. DUMC Photography.

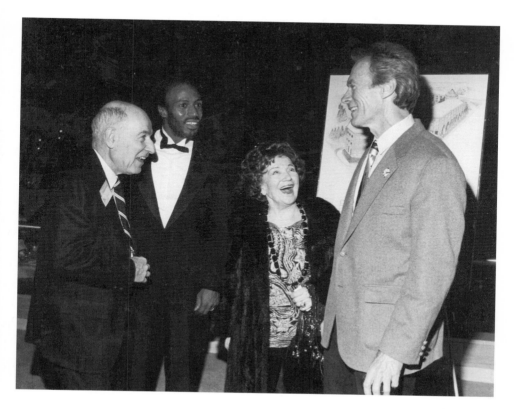

5 Clint Eastwood and Thelonius Monk visiting Duke Medical Center to consider establishing the Thelonius Monk Institute of Jazz, with Ella Fountain Pratt, Durham, January 1989. DUMC Photography.

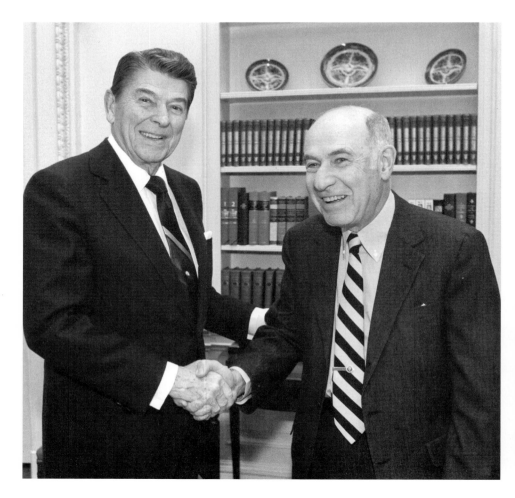

6   Dr. W. G. Anlyan meeting President Ronald Reagan in the Oval Room on the occasion of the conclusion of his term on the President's Science Advisory Council, January 13, 1989. From personal archive of author.

THE WHITE HOUSE

WASHINGTON

January 11, 1989

Dear Dr. Anlyan:

As my Administration comes to a close, I want to thank you for
your contributions to national policy for science and technology.
A true measure of responsible citizenship is one's willingness to
make personal and professional sacrifices in the national interest.
By your efforts on the White House Science Council you have
done a great service for your country -- and done so without
fanfare or wide public recognition. But one of the reasons the
Council has been so successful in helping shape Federal policy
for science, technology, and national defense has been its ability
to deliberate thoughtfully and quietly and then provide expert
advice directly to the people making decisions. We deeply
appreciate that dedication.

Nancy and I wish you continued success in all your future
endeavors, and we convey the Nation's heartfelt thanks for a
job well done.

Sincerely,

Ronald Reagan

Dr. William Anlyan
Chancellor
Duke University
Post Office Box 3701
Durham, North Carolina 27710

7   Letter of appreciation from President
Reagan. DUMC Photography.

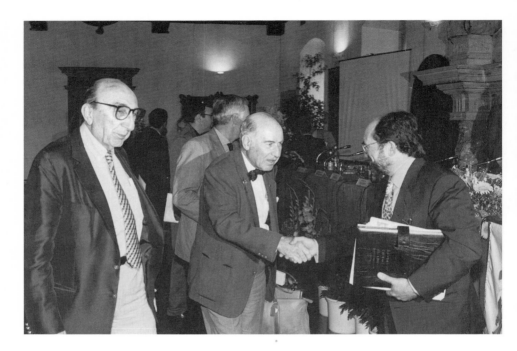

8   Dr. Michael DeBakey and Dr. Mario E. Bianchetti Castel Madruzzo at the European Health Care System Conference held in Milan and Trento, Italy, to discuss programs to unify medical education programs in Europe, 1992. From personal archive of author.

9

BUILDING FOR EXCELLENCE

GROWTH DEPENDS ON planning sensibly for the needs of the future. The simplest example would be to build a parking deck, taking into consideration the projected growth in parking needs: you have to plan for reasonable need and propitious use of the facility without overbuilding. Also, in planning for future needs, one has to be careful to make sure that not only the necessary capital funds for expansion are there but also the funds for operating and maintaining the quality of the building. Unfortunately, at Duke University Medical Center we have always been three to five years behind in meeting our needs.

In terms of growth in programs, such as the number of medical students per class, one has to look at factors such as the number of highly qualified applicants; the facilities that would support the teaching programs, including libraries, auditoriums, and laboratories; and the need for small-group instruction. Careful planning is extremely important, and I was fortunate to have inherited Lou Swanson as physical planner from my predecessor, Barnes Woodhall. Along with Charlie Frenzel, Lou Swanson was key in planning the 1957 expansion of the hospital. Subsequently, Dr. Woodhall depended heavily on his planning abilities.

When I came along, it was obvious we needed not only a physical planning arm but also a program planning arm. I was very fortunate in being able to recruit Dr. Jane Elchlepp, who was equally adept at programmatic and physical planning.

I had always been mystified by how Tom Kinney, with a very extensive out-of-town program, could return to Durham late one night, yet be in

my office at 7:30 the next morning with complete plans drawn up for the
expansion of the Department of Pathology. I found out later that Dr. Elchlepp in his department was the person who did all the leg work; she briefed
Dr. Kinney just before he saw me, and Dr. Kinney was marvelous at sound-
ing as though he had been part of the planning process right from the
ground up. I asked Dr. Kinney if I could sign up Dr. Elchlepp for one-third
of her time, and he very graciously agreed. A few months later, Dr. Elchlepp came to see me and said that there must be some misunderstanding,
because she thought one-third of her time was one-third of eight hours a
day and not one-third of twenty-four hours a day. To be correct, she spent
ten to twelve hours a day at her job with me.

Jane was a tall, athletic woman with a fondness for Navajo jewelry; she
looked like the Westerner she was. She had been a schoolteacher in Saint
Louis when she was discovered by Dr. Jane Philpott—who later came to
Duke as a professor of botany—who thought that she was underemployed
for her capabilities. This was very true, because subsequently she managed
to combine teaching at Roosevelt College in Chicago with obtaining a doc-
torate in pathology at the University of Chicago. She impressed her Ph.D.
mentors to the extent that they persuaded her to go on and get an M.D.
Thereafter, she specialized in pathology, but because she was not wealthy
and came from a family of limited means, she joined the Public Health Service. By our good fortune she was assigned to the Department of Pathology
at Duke under Wiley Forbus, where I first met her.

Jane was a genius. She could talk to architects, engineers, and all kinds of
computer specialists in their own language and at their own level. She could
also talk to bricklayers with authority because she was a member of the
bricklayers union. Each one of them had the utmost respect for her abilities.
They called her Lady Jane. She was the backbone of planning for many of
the facilities that were constructed during my time at Duke, including the
Seeley G. Mudd Building and particularly the new hospital (which would
be known as the North Division, to differentiate it from the old hospital,
henceforth called the South Division). She did a magnificent job, along
with Lou Swanson and Larry Nelson, who subsequently joined them as the
in-house architect; and before that she had Wally Jarboe, a retired Air Force
colonel who had specialized in supervising hospital construction, on her
team. Jane coordinated all of this, and most of the time I would go along
with her suggestions. On some rare occasions I would disagree for reasons
that she did not have the background to know. I don't think we could have
done anywhere near the job we did without Jane's input and teamwork.

She was quiet, self-effacing, did not exalt her talents, and gained the respect of all the top chairmen in the Medical Center. My only major disagreement with her was when I insisted on doubling the size of the women's restroom in the new Searle Center. I did not want to have the embarrassing scene of women waiting in line outside their facility.

The original Duke Medical School and Hospital were Wilburt Davison's brainchild, and the wonderful thing about them was that the doors of the Medical School opened onto the main university campus. That set the scene for the Medical Center as part of the larger university, not as a separate entity across town or in another community. In addition, the hospital and laboratories—the clinical and basic science components of the Medical School, respectively—were all pulled together, because a medical education takes place not only in labs and classrooms, but also at the patients' bedsides.

Construction on the Medical School and hospital began in 1927, and both opened for business in 1930. Additional construction began almost immediately, with the building of Baker House, the nurses' dormitory in 1931, and a library reading room in 1934. There were major expansions of the hospital in 1940 and 1957, adding approximately two hundred beds, outpatient areas, and operating rooms. Dr. Davison was the prime mover in both cases. There was also a certain amount of expansion of the hospital to the south and north, with the addition of the Deryl Hart Pavilion, Diagnostic and Treatment Building I (D&TR I) for hematology in 1956, D&TR II for radiation therapy in 1959, and D&TR III in 1960. The diagnostic and treatment buildings were largely made possible by funds released by the Hill-Burton Act. Since the funds generated by private practice supported in large measure the finances of the respective clinical department, more beds meant more income. The competition among the clinical departments for the allocation of beds was very aggressive.

By the time the nurses' dormitory was moved out of Baker House to the newly constructed Hanes House, we had run out of land needed for further contiguous growth—the contiguity that had been one of the hallmarks of Duke's Medical Center. Another problem, in terms of the Medical Center as a whole, was that the departments that had moneys to ante up put it in a pot to help fund expansion; thus, surgery and medicine, the richest departments, got the lion's share of the new additions, and the basic sciences, pediatrics, and other less affluent departments got much less new space. It was not a well-balanced distribution of space, and this inequity—as some see it—has bedeviled the Medical Center throughout its history.

There was one noncontiguous Medical Center building early on, and that was the original Bell Building, which stood literally in the woods of the 9,000-odd-acre Duke Forest. The forest came down almost to the gravel parking lot in front of the original hospital. The university trustees decreed that if any brick building were to be built—a building not in the Gothic style nor of the gray Duke stone that characterize the university as well as the early hospital and Medical School buildings—it would have to be built beyond what Duke trustees called the "green belt," in the woods. That is why Part 1 of Bell Building, built in 1944 out of the desperate need for research space that could not be accommodated in the Davison Building, was built of lowly red brick. As more money became available, a cross-wing was built onto Bell, and then another cross-wing, until today the Bell Building has five parts.

My first brush with Medical Center construction came in my internship year, and Dr. Davison was the instigator. It was shortly after I came here, when we lived near that winding one-lane Erwin Road that disappeared into the Duke Forest. Bulldozers appeared about a block away and flattened a large expanse of land, changing the course of Erwin Road. I remember taking my oldest child walking on Sunday afternoons to see the holes that the bulldozers had created. There, the Veterans Administration Hospital was to be built; today it represents an important part of the greater Duke Medical Center.

The construction of Hanes House in 1951, replacing Baker House as a home and dormitory for student nurses, was the next project in which I had an interest. Baker House had been separate from the old hospital building and is the only building on the Medical Center campus that is not in line with other buildings, going by floor levels. The floor-to-ceiling heights in Baker House are much lower than those in the hospital, because in 1930 no one thought Baker House would ever be connected to the rest of the Medi-cal Center. Yet in 1940 when the new addition—the PDC building—was built, it became necessary to connect the hospital to Baker House. Ramps were built to make for a more or less smooth connection.

When Baker House was evacuated by the nurses, a grab-as-grab-can situation ensued, chiefly between the Department of Medicine and the De-partment of Surgery. All sorts of games were played, with various com-ponents of the departments being moved into the building to establish squatters' rights. Everyone stayed away from the second and third floors, which it was agreed should become rooms for the house staff who re-mained on call. Up to that time, house staff had slept in odd rooms all over the Medical Center in non-air-conditioned, very tight quarters and bunks. The components of surgical faculty offices that went to Baker House were neurosurgery, plastic surgery, and some general surgery; medicine had neurology, and Dr. Stead's office.

Another building project with which I became involved was the Diagnostic and Treatment Building III in 1960. In particular, I was interested in the design of the new laboratories and offices that Dr. Hart had assigned to me. Up to that time I had had a small office next to Dr. Hart's office, between Halsted and McDowell wards in the main hospital, and the room across the hall where my secretary resided. It was wonderful to be able to design an entirely new office suite and laboratory. By that time it had become apparent that Donald Silver would join me in the laboratory as a senior staff member, so I cut the size of my office in half to create an office for Dr. Silver. He took over my research program after I accepted the deanship.

Thus the Medical Center had grown over the years, but it had been more or less a random process. By the time Barnes Woodhall became dean of the Medical School in 1960, it was evident that the growth of the Medical Center needed to be planned in a more logical manner.

In 1960 Dr. Woodhall hired the Chicago consultants Booz, Allen & Hamilton to do a programmatic study of what was needed; they in turn subcontracted the architectural planning to Todd Wheeler, Perkins & Will, another Chicago firm. Together, these consultants laid the plans for the systematic expansion of the Medical Center. After the two studies were completed, Dr. Woodhall took the results to Duke's Board of Trustees, who allocated eighty acres of land to the Medical Center, which were to provide for our northward expansion for the foreseeable future. As it turned out, we covered up the land in less than thirty years.

During my tenure, the need—and the means—for constructing additional facilities were prodigious. I was responsible for all of the construction beginning with the animal farm buildings in 1965, going through the North Division of Duke University Hospital, the Seeley G. Mudd Building, the Bryan Neurobiology Building, and all the research buildings that were completed by or shortly after 1989. Construction costs were roughly $288 million. (Replacement costs in 1999 were estimated at $642 million.) In all, we added more than 1.6 million square feet of space.

National, regional, and local factors worked in our favor. Above all, there was the strong economy that followed World War II, unlike the recessionary times the country had seen after World War I. This helped make possible the ambitious generosity of the NIH, funding great research initiatives, and the Hill-Burton Act, which promoted the construction of clinical facilities. By this time, also, the South finally partook of the nation's prosperity. North Carolina, in particular, benefited from the far-sighted policies of people such as Governor Terry Sanford, who promoted the development of an effective road system throughout the state and fostered a much wider-ranging educational system than seen before, making higher education accessible to almost all who wanted it.

At the Medical Center we had an ambitious, very active faculty, which in turn attracted an ever higher quality of students. Duke's fairly centralized Medical Center administration gave wide latitude to the department chair, yet we also could plan for the institution as a whole, making reasonable plans that had every chance of succeeding. The ever far-sighted Barnes Woodhall was also among the first—if not the first—medical dean to establish a planning office, which opened in 1962 with Louis Swanson and Bill Reed as its first staffers. We had the support of The Duke Endowment, which has the continuing well-being of Duke University in all its manifestations as one of its major purposes. Then, too, we have been able to count on the generous help of alumni, grateful patients, and people who simply are willing to support the best that medicine can provide in its time.

And so the Medical Center was developed in a northward direction toward Erwin Road and, not so incidentally, toward the Durham VA Hospital. The research facilities line a road now called Science Drive.

An exception to that northward thrust was the animal farm. When I first came to Duke, and for a long period thereafter, animals were housed in the basement of the Bell Building and in the attic of the Davison Building under what we today would call primitive, inadequate conditions. At the peak of my own research career, around 1961, my laboratory had the largest collection of experimental dogs in the institution, and we kept them in both places. In 1965, to provide better facilities for the animals, we converted one of the old Duke properties into an animal farm so that for long-term studies the dogs would not have to be in small cages but would have greater freedom to roam. The cost of maintaining the animals this way was much lower, while the conditions for them were much better.

It then became apparent that we needed to build a vivarium, a place where experimental animals could be kept in the acute phase of a study, as opposed to the long-term phase, where one can put them out on the farm. I learned that the rules and regulations for housing animals in the acute stage are much more complex than the rules for building a hospital for humans. With the help of some NIH guidelines and money, we built an ultramodern facility. We only had one problem: we had some infections early on. These had occurred—as Jane Elchlepp, of the planning and construction team, discovered—because a duct from one of the toilets went through the sterile animal air supply system. We quickly corrected the plumbing.

Through the years, we have had periodic challenges from various animal rights groups, but fortunately we have not attracted any of the controversy that our neighbor, the University of North Carolina in Chapel Hill, has faced. Nevertheless, I think we in the research field ought to be more concerned about experimental animals than anyone else, and treat the animals better than anyone else could, given the circumstances.

The Vivarium came from a special fund available for animal facilities, and thanks to the Cancer Act passed in 1971, some matching funds became available from the National Cancer Institute; these helped pay for the construction of both the Jones Building for basic cancer research and the Animal Laboratory Isolation Facility in 1975, as well as the Morris Building for the clinical cancer programs in 1978. After that, our construction costs were covered completely by private funds.

The first building in which I had a major involvement was the Nanaline Duke Building, which was completed in 1968. With this building we tapped some of the last bits of federal money available for the construction of basic science facilities. Dan Tosteson had been the major workhorse in writing the NIH application for this research facility. The NIH funding game was a highly competitive one, and the strength of our proposals was always the programmatic content, not beautiful architecture. Architecture was a consideration, however. The unit cost of the building had to be reasonable, and sometimes during site visits we were questioned about our use of Duke stone, which was slightly more expensive than brick or wood would have been. We always called it the "Duke gargoyle factor," though we did not put gargoyles on any of those Medical Center buildings (they are only on the Davison Building). The Duke stone, which distinguishes the buildings on Duke's West Campus, including Duke Chapel, is a beautiful one, but it has two drawbacks: the Hillsborough quarry eleven miles away that furnishes it is coming to the end of its supply, and thus the stone is becoming more difficult and costly to quarry; in addition, there are fewer and fewer stonemasons and their services, too, are becoming more expensive. In buildings constructed now, Duke stone is used as a decorative element rather than as the basic building material. I think in the long run the slight additional expense has paid off, because we don't have a series of incompatible architectural facades; they blend into one another.

The Nanaline Duke Building was the first major departure from contiguity. Up to that point, additions to the Medical Center, except for the Bell Building, had always managed to be pasted onto the existing Davison Building/Duke Hospital complex. As might be expected, to move from the traditional way of doing things entailed a hard-fought battle, but it was a necessity. Having all of the medical programs under one roof is a convenience when getting from point A to point B, especially in rain or snow, but it became an impossibility as the Medical Center population grew from the hundreds to the thousands.

We did create contiguity of a sort for the research complex that was subsequently constructed: every building in the complex—the Nanaline Duke Building, the Alex H. Sands Building, the Edwin A. Jones Building and the others that followed—are connected by walkways to their neighboring buildings. It also became apparent when we moved the basic scientists from the Bell Building to the Nanaline Duke Building that they missed the interaction with their clinical research colleagues, who had also been in the Bell Building (mixing basic and clinical scientists is what we call the "Bell Building phenomenon"). In subsequent projects, we made sure not only that the research buildings were physically connected but that each complex housed a mix of clinical and basic scientists.

The Alex H. Sands Building of 1973 was the second major basic science building to be developed on the new research campus. It was particularly important, when we sought to bring Dave Robertson aboard as the new chairman of anatomy, to have some research facilities for that field, including cell biology and neurobiology. Dr. Robertson himself was a basic neurobiologist. I was able to put together enough private moneys, with a match from The Duke Endowment, to support the construction of the building. It was named for Alex Sands, vice chairman of The Duke Endowment for many years and a person on whom the leadership of the Endowment, including Mr. Duke, had relied. The name was suggested by Dick Henney, who was both a trustee and the executive director of The Duke Endowment.

The Edwin A. Jones Building (1976) came about shortly after I recruited Bill Joklik to head microbiology and immunology; at the same time, the cancer program had gotten a financial and psychological boost from President Nixon's "war on cancer" and was ready to become a comprehensive cancer center. In our planning we felt that we would need two facilities — one for basic cancer research; the other, somewhere in the clinical complex, devoted to the care of cancer patients.

The lead gift for the Jones Building, the basic cancer research facility, came from Duke trustee Edwin Jones Jr., his family, and his corporation, in honor of Edwin Jones Sr., who had also been a trustee and a member of the building and grounds committee. Edwin Jones Sr. in his day was CEO of the J. A. Jones Construction Company, which was founded by his father. The senior Ed Jones was the contractor who built Oak Ridge, especially the purification center for uranium. It is said that there were only three people who had a complete picture of why Oak Ridge was being built during World War II: President Roosevelt, Major General Leslie Groves, and Edwin Jones Sr. Even Vice President Truman did not know about Oak Ridge until he became president. About $4.4 million for the Jones Building came from the National Cancer Institute; the rest of the money was raised from private sources.

The clinical component of the Duke Comprehensive Cancer Center is the Edwin A. Morris Building, named for one of our grateful cancer patients, who made the lead gift of $1 million toward its construction. John Thomas, of the center's development staff, was very helpful in working with Ed Morris. About $4.2 million came from the NIH, and much of the credit for raising the rest of the funding goes to Bill Shingleton, at that time director of the Duke Comprehensive Cancer Center.

In 1969 we built the Marshall I. Pickens Building. There was money available at that time from governmental resources for rehabilitation medicine. Duke at the time had no such program, and we had hoped that by erecting this building, we would create a focal point for rehabilitation medicine. There were two trends in the world of rehabilitation at that time. One was the model followed at New York University and at Northwestern University in Chicago, where physical medicine/rehabilitation was a separate department. The individuals running those two units made them outstanding, but other rehabilitation units around the country were second- or third-rate. The same could be said of some of the VA hospitals where departments of physical medicine/rehabilitation have become traditional. The alternative model, which prevailed at Duke, was to have the burdens of rehabilitation borne by orthopedics, plastic surgery, and neurology, with the help of physical therapy, but under the care of a physician specialist interested in rehabilitation. We chose to stay with the latter model, which has been quite successful at Duke. In contrast, at the VA across the street from Duke, physical medicine/rehabilitation had been relatively weak.

Marshall Pickens was chairman of the board of The Duke Endowment at that time. A Duke alumnus and long-time supporter of the Medical Center, he was also on the executive committee of the Duke University Board of Trustees. We thought it would be fitting to honor him by putting his name on the building. Getting the money from the endowment for this building was not contingent on the naming of the building—the building was named to honor a man who had served the university and Medical Center well. Subsequently, when rehabilitation didn't fly as a separate unit, we converted the building to a primary care center, and when the Department of Community and Family Medicine was formed, we assigned most of the space to that department.

By the late sixties the need for research space had become critical; there was no way we could get enough space fast enough to hold onto our outstanding research faculty. We thought of putting up temporary buildings, much as they had at Oxford University around the old Radcliffe Infirmary, but we knew that the university trustees would not permit unsightly temporary structures. They certainly would not allow us to have trailers parked on the campus. Thanks to the ingenuity of my colleague Jane Elchlepp, we came up with the term "limited-life building," and we went on to build four of them surrounding the Vivarium. The limited-life buildings—also known as Research Park 1, 2, 3, and 4—went up in 1969 and 1970, and over thirty years later are still holding up very well.

The Civitan Building represented a great deal of hard work by Bud Busse, chairman of psychiatry, and his staff, working with the Civitan organization. The building was the brainchild of one of the developmental psychiatrists, who saw the need for a regional resource to study and treat the developmental problems of children. There were similar centers in other parts of the country, but none had worked out well. During this period the government had a special interest in the developmental problems of children, spurred on by the involvement of President Kennedy and his family in view of the problems of Rosemary Kennedy, the president's sister. The Kennedy Foundation was providing support for initiatives in this area, and Dr. Busse hoped to tap into these funds. However, after President Kennedy was shot, the foundation declined and so, of course, did the Kennedy influence. Dr. Busse received a grant of $100,000 from the Civitans, who recognized the need for such a resource, but finding funding was a continuing problem. When the building was finally constructed in 1970–71, we could only finish one floor; the second floor came later. The child development center never did get off the ground, in spite of the work of Dr. Busse and his staff and the cooperation of the Department of Pediatrics. Today the Civitan Building houses various programs in psychiatry. Not all good ideas work out successfully.

The Duke Eye Center was developed in fulfillment of a promise to Joe Wadsworth when he was recruited as chairman of ophthalmology. Dr. Wadsworth was key to raising much of the funding for the building, which was constructed in 1973.

One of the embarrassments of Duke University Medical Center had long been that the Medical Center library was in an enclosed courtyard in the Davison Building, with 60 percent of our holdings in storage in warehouses on the campus. A new Medical Center library was a very high priority in my book. We could not achieve being a top-flight medical school without a respectable medical library and information resource. In the master plan, we had intended to site the building on the hill where the coal pile from the West Campus heating plant is located, because the university in the sixties had planned to go to an all-electric campus. (Some members of Duke's trustees also served on the boards of The Duke Endowment and the Duke Power Company. In essence we were planning an all-electric campus because of advice about the future of energy resources. But then in the seventies the price of electricity soared, and it became obvious that it would be more economical to retain the steam plant generated by coal.) Therefore, the Medical Center library was built in 1975 in the valley where it is now located, 150 or so yards beyond the "coal pile" between the South and North Divisions of Duke Hospital.

Fortunately for us, the Seeley G. Mudd Fund was looking for opportunities to fund special buildings on university and college campuses. We invited the then head of the foundation, Robert D. Fisher, to come to Duke on a visit with his wife, and persuaded him to put $1.5 million into the building. Dr. Martin Cummings, a Duke alumnus and then director of the National Library of Medicine, emphasized that the future was uncertain with regard to the balance of books vis-à-vis other communications media, and we followed his suggestion to leave the space flexible so we could accommodate whatever the future might bring (and has, indeed, brought). I also persuaded the clinical chairmen to commit about $850,000 toward the building, which they did reluctantly and only after I threatened to withhold approval from other construction projects closer to their hearts.

Despite these commitments, we were still shy of the sum needed to develop the entire building, which was fortuitous. We had left the ground-level area as a shell as the library took shape in 1975, anticipating that some day we might put an auditorium there. In January 1977 Dan and Bill Searle and their brother-in-law, Wes Dixon, came to visit me. At that time, I was on the board of the G. D. Searle Pharmaceutical Company. They were anxious to recruit Don Rumsfeld, who had been President Ford's chief of staff, as the new Searle CEO, and they were visiting all external board members to acquaint them with the opportunity. While they were on the Duke campus I took them to the Seeley G. Mudd Building, showed them the shell space, and told them that for a contribution of $1 million we could finish it up as a continuing education center for the health sciences and name it for the Searle family. The suggestion was made off the cuff, and I would not have been surprised if they had declined, given the amount I requested rather brashly. However, they called me within two weeks and told me they would make the contribution of $1 million. As it was, finishing the shell space cost only around $800,000, so we put the rest of the money into an endowment fund for the operation of the building.

The whole idea for the layout of the Searle Center came to me through the many AAMC meetings I attended in the lower levels of the Washington Hilton Hotel, where a large open space with movable walls and small meeting rooms on the perimeter make meetings of all sizes possible. This was the pattern followed in the Searle Center. There also are kitchen facilities so that excellent food can be served—warm.

Through Jane Elchlepp, we hired Durham architect Max Isley for the work on the Searle Center. I told him at the outset that this area was going to be designed starting with the crystal chandeliers—from ceiling to floor, not the other way around. When he realized I was not kidding, I was flooded with catalogs of chandeliers. I learned more about chandeliers than I ever cared to know. I picked chandeliers as symbols of elegance—to mark this as a place where we could finally entertain visitors in style; it was part of my plan to sell people on what a great place Duke University Medical Center is. Until the Searle Center opened, we had held our dinners, luncheons, and meetings in rather shabby second-hand places; we did not have an elegant spot on the entire campus. For instance, when Dr. Sabiston had a meeting of one of the distinguished surgical societies, he had to get in line to use the second-floor dining room of the university's Union Building, and then he had to put Oriental rugs on the floor to make it look at least somewhat elegant.

As the years went by and some of the key people at the Medical Center began to die, it became obvious that we had no appropriate place to put their ashes. The entrance of the Davison Building had been reserved for the ashes of the original chairmen and deans, but those entrance walls were pretty well filled up. I created a "cemetery," or columbarium, along the main hall of the Searle Center, with the proviso that chairmen and deans be on the right-hand wall, and division heads and other distinguished faculty and staff on the left-hand wall. It soon became apparent that the demand for this columbarium was going to be very extensive over the decades, so we asked Larry Nelson, the Duke Medical Center architect, to design the rest of the corridors to hold even more urns. I never thought I'd be running a cemetery. I've reserved my spot, right between Barnes Woodhall and Tom Kinney, where some of my ashes will rest between two of my dearest colleagues and mentors.

The Searle Center opened in 1978 and has become a useful part of the Medical Center community as well as all components of the university, serving countless thousands each year. Elegant dinners for 250 are regular events, receptions for 900 are handled routinely—and at Christmas time, there are two parties for 5,000 each (one for the Medical Center day staff, one for the night staff).

When we were constructing the first parking deck, around 1972, Lou Swanson came to see me. He told me that two levels would take care of the parking situation for the foreseeable future. I told him that he was going to build three levels because I didn't want to hear about parking for a while. As it turned out, within six months the three levels were pretty full most of the time, and parking—or the lack thereof—continues to be one of the issues facing the Medical Center.

Planning for a new hospital building started with Barnes Woodhall around 1962, when it became apparent that we were never going to get out of the bind of inadequate clinical facilities by enclosing more courtyards or adding another bump, as had been done in 1957 with what has become part of the Deryl Hart Pavilion. Dr. Woodhall as well as the consultants—Booz, Allen & Hamilton—got a lot of faculty involved in the planning process. Unfortunately, the project did not move along, and many of the faculty were disappointed with what turned out to be a futile exercise. So when I became dean in 1964, one of the lessons I had learned from the previous deliberations was not to mobilize people in a program that was not going to come to fruition any time soon. In the meantime, the Woodhall Building—known as the main entrance building—had been built, and it gave relief to two of the most hard-pressed areas in the hospital, obstetrics-gynecology and psychiatry. In addition, the federally funded Clinical Research Unit was established in one of the D&TR buildings; the CRU is where clinical studies requiring exceptionally rigorous controls are carried out. The immediate terrible pressure was off, but the long-term needs were growing.

About 1971 I began to feel that the time had come to consider building a new hospital. Obviously, this would be a substantial undertaking, and it was extremely fortunate that the university president at the time was Terry Sanford and that the chairman of the board was Alexander McMahon, president of the American Hospital Association. Both of them were big thinkers and not afraid of major projects. With the help of the staff, and especially with Jane Elchlepp and Lou Swanson, we acquired the services of Perkins & Will. In 1972 we got the concurrence of the executive committee of the Duke University Board of Trustees to proceed with more detailed planning.

A site was selected: the area north of the original hospital, on Erwin Road. Hence it became the North Division of Duke University Hospital. We considered two major alternatives: one was to build a partial replacement of the old hospital, the other was to build a total replacement. As I recall, the total replacement would have cost $150 million, whereas the partial replacement—leaving ob-gyn and psychiatry in the existing hospital and somehow connecting the two buildings—was around $95 million. A total new structure would have been smoother, but I already had a lot of objections on the part of the clinical staff, who thought it was folly spending $95 million on a structure so far away from the existing hospital. However, with the support of my staff and President Sanford, Alex McMahon, and especially Henry Rauch, who was vice chairman of the Duke University Board of Trustees and chairman of the Medical Center's Board of Visitors, we persuaded the trustees to go ahead with the $95 million project. Some of the trustees were shocked at the size of the project. It was bigger than anything—including the rest of the total university—that they had previously approved. But Mr. Rauch backed the project, and he was very persuasive; his condition was that we be able to raise $40 million of the $95 million— the rest was feasible with a private placement of bonds. At that time, we did not have the N.C. hospital bond issue; that was something we worked on after the hospital was built. Once the N.C. hospital bond issue was approved by the state legislature and the governor, we converted from private funding to public funding.

To make up 40 percent of the costs with gifts, I approached The Duke

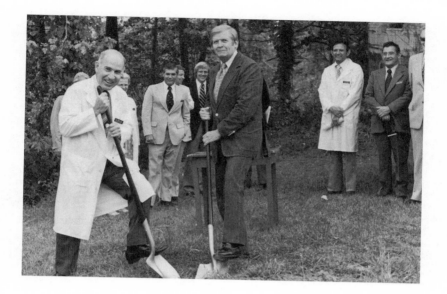

16　Ground breaking for Duke Hospital North with President
Terry Sanford, September 1975. DUMC Photography.

Endowment for $10 million over a period of years, which they approved.
I asked the building fund of the medical and surgical PDCs for $5 million;
I also asked the clinical departments to subscribe another $5 million from
their clinical reserves, on the basis that medicine and surgery would put
in $2 million a piece and the extra $1 million would come from the other
clinical departments in proportion to the contributions they made to the
building fund. Obviously, the clinical departments were going to be the
beneficiaries of the new hospital, which would generate more income for
them. They concurred. Some of the clinical faculty referred to the hospital
project as "Anlyan's folly," and I am not sure that the project would have
been approved had I put the matter to a vote of the clinical faculty. Nevertheless, I decided to go ahead with the project. It was one of the few times
I had to proceed undemocratically.

We had some interesting twists in the planning process. I remember
in particular the intervention of two trustees. One was George McGhee,
former U.S. ambassador to Turkey. He had been a patient at the National
Cancer Institute, having been housed during his radical neck surgery in the
clinical center at NIH. He was impressed with the fact that the whole clinical

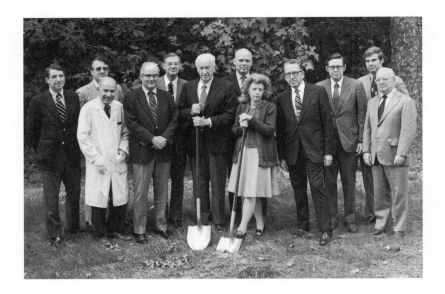

17 Trustees of The Duke Endowment at the ground breaking for Duke Hospital North. DUMC Photography.

center had semiprivate rooms, although he was never told that the facility was maintained at 50 percent occupancy so as to give every patient, who was nominally in a semiprivate room, in actual fact a large private room. He voiced the opinion that if we built semiprivate rooms in Duke North instead of single rooms (which is what we did build), we would halve the costs. The other trustee who gave me a bit of a time was the former CEO of Montgomery Ward, Ed Donnell, who insisted that the most heat- and air-conditioning-efficient buildings for Montgomery Ward were square or rectangular, without understanding the fact that the fire and safety rules for hospitals specify that every patient room has to have an exterior window. At any event, we engaged the services of Hellmuth, Obata & Kassebaum out of Saint Louis, the firm that had designed the National Air and Space Museum in Washington. Gyo Obata was the design architect who developed the North Division of Duke University Hospital. We started the construction in 1975, and it was completed on schedule and on budget in 1980.

One side issue was establishing a transportation system between the two hospital buildings, which are about 1,200 feet apart. Three companies competed to provide the transport system. One was Westinghouse, which had put in the connecting system at Hartsfield Airport in Atlanta; the second was the corporation that put in the connector at the Dallas–Fort Worth airport and that went defunct shortly after; and the third was Otis. Otis was a highly respected name in the vertical transport business but new in horizontal transportation. It so happened that Dr. Sabiston and I were in Colorado Springs at the American Surgical Association meeting just about the time the matter was under consideration, and we flew up to Denver to look at the Otis system that was on a test track outside the city. One of the impressive things about the system was that it blew the snow as it moved, so that the snow in Denver was not a problem for the horizontal movement of the transport system. What we did not factor in was that snow in Denver is dry powder snow, and that snow in North Carolina tends to be wet and ice rather quickly, as we subsequently learned. In any event, the Otis people won the competition, which was carefully examined by Jane Elchlepp and a group of consultants. Even after we had chosen Otis, university trustee Edward Jones Jr. asked whether we should not reexamine the Westinghouse proposal. I believe he had been lobbied fairly extensively by the Westinghouse people, who had not given up. So the whole issue was reexamined, with more consultants, and more trustees, and the Otis choice was upheld. The winning part of the Otis proposal was that the system would not have to stay on the same level with reference to sea level, it could go slightly up or down (i.e., travel underground to Parking Deck II, a connection that was contemplated but never actually completed), in contrast to the Westinghouse system, which had to be all on one level. Unfortunately, Otis was subsequently bought up by United Technology, and they separated the firm's vertical transport component from the horizontal transport division, and we were afraid at one time that they would go defunct as well. Thanks to the persistence of Jane Elchlepp and her staff, and a lot of legal help, we were able to maintain the system. The PRT (personal rapid transport) system that is in place now transports patients, faculty, staff, and visitors from one division of the hospital to the other in approximately seventy seconds. The trains move on the Hovercraft principle, traveling on one-quarter inch of air and propelled along by linear induction motors. Parallel to the PRT tracks is a walkway for those who prefer—and are able—to cover the distance between the two sections of Duke University Hospital on foot. There is also a "drawbridge" that goes up and thus interrupts the PRT traffic whenever a train comes to deliver more coal for the large black

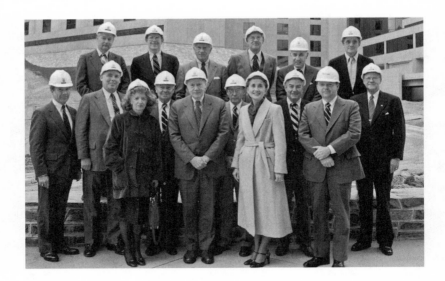

18   Trustees of The Duke Endowment visiting the construction site of the new Duke Hospital North. Among those present are (front row, L–R) Mary Semans, Archie Davis (chairman of the Board of Trustees), Juanita Kreps, Chancellor Ken Pye of Duke University. DUMC Photography.

pile looming just to the west of the tracks. Here the twenty-first century meets the nineteenth century.

With the North Division, we also brought in another form of transportation: helicopter service. Duke was probably one of the first major hospitals to provide such a service as a routine matter. I remember in 1961, when we were planning what is now the Woodhall Building, I was a young surgeon responsible for planning the new emergency room to replace the two-room facility in the Davison Building. With a committee I designed what would be latest and best in emergency rooms, 1961 edition, and as part of that, I advocated putting a heliport on top of the Woodhall Building. I received no support from the administration. Among the other reasons, I remember Lou Swanson of the planning office saying it would be a fire hazard for the building. I had even gone so far as to have the elevators in the Woodhall Building designed so that they could have functioned from the roof down, if the heliport had been put in. So when the new hospital was being built between 1975 and 1980, I insisted that we plan on helicopter service. We came to a final decision in the early 1980s. For some reason the hospital administration was opposed to it because it would not be cost-effective. I persuaded them that we should put it in because that was the way of the future, even if it was going to be a loss-leader. In looking around for helicopter companies, the successful bidder was the company of Buddy Schoellkopf, the former husband of Caroline Hunt of Dallas, and a formal helicopter service was inaugurated. The heliport is adjacent to the emergency room of Duke North so that patients can be wheeled in quickly. I had a little bit of trouble with one of the Durham City Council members, the wife of a Duke English professor, who vetoed it on one occasion on the basis that it would be used by me personally to speed up the transit time between the Medical Center and Raleigh-Durham airport. It gave me a taste of the stupidity in politics. Incidentally, the helicopter service has been highly successful, used not only to speed accident victims to the hospital, which is what we had originally thought would be the main use, but also to bring cardiac patients in from the surrounding area for immediate care. As we now know, this is vital in determining the outcome of many such events. There are now three landing pads outside the North Division.

One other side issue was the red-brick Bell Building. Situated between the two gray stone hospitals, it stuck out like the proverbial sore thumb. That problem was solved by painting the Bell Building a color that would not clash in appearance with the new hospital. After seeing the newly painted structure, some of our older faculty could not believe that it was the same old Bell Building.

The North Division consists essentially of two buildings. One is the patient tower, which contained 616 patient rooms when it opened (there have been several additions to the bed count over the years), and the central circulation core, that is, elevators and stairs. This is the "hotel" of the hospital. Attached to it is a large, lower building that contains the "working" parts of the hospital: a large diagnostic radiology suite, including a number of magnetic resonance imaging scanners; a twenty-nine-room operating suite; pharmacy; and laboratories; and the large emergency/trauma suite, immediately adjacent to the heliport. A dedicated elevator stands ready at all times to move patients from the emergency room to the operating room suite. The North Division houses the inpatient units for medicine, surgery, pediatrics, and obstetrics-gynecology. A separate children's hospital has just opened adjacent to the North Division. This allows outpatient pediatrics to connect directly with the fifth floor pediatric inpatient unit in the North Division, thus consolidating the care of children to one geographic location.

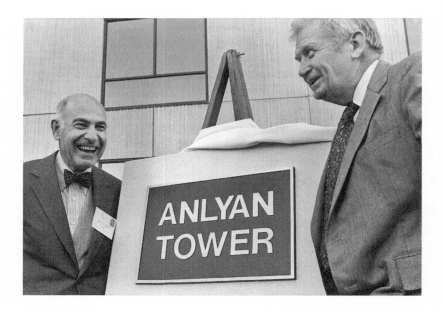

19   Dr. W. G. Anlyan with President Sanford at the unveiling of the plaque to be fixed to the front wall of Duke Hospital North, November 11, 1983. DUMC Photography.

One of the outstanding features of the North Division is that while the bed tower has a standard twelve-foot floor-to-floor height, the ancillary building is constructed with a twenty-four-foot floor-to-floor height. It allows interstitial spaces between the floors, so that changes to the many electrical, gas, and other systems that are part of medical care and that inevitably change in our fast-moving technological world, can be made without disrupting the functions on the floors above and below.

The final major building during my years as head of the Medical Center was the Joseph and Kathleen Bryan Research Building for Neurobiology, which opened in 1990. Several events led up to the construction of this building. For almost ten years I had felt that our school of medicine needed a neurobiology department. It seemed to me more reasonable to look at organ-related departments of the future, namely, cell biology and neurobiology, rather than the older basic sciences of physiology and anatomy. With that partly in mind, I was looking for other areas of strength within neurobiology, both basic and clinical. About that time neurologist Allen Roses

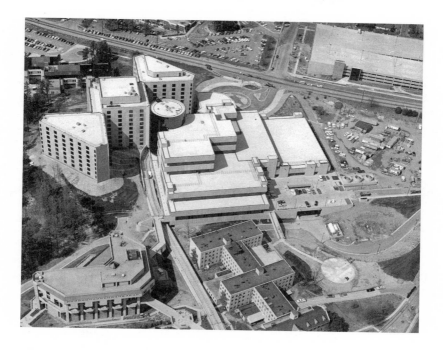

20   Aerial photograph of Duke Hospital
North. DUMC Photography.

was beginning to investigate the bases of some kinds of Alzheimer's disease. I had originally interested Allen in Alzheimer's when the NIH issued a request for proposals; up to then he had had no interest in that disease whatsoever. I invited him to my office one day and said, "Allen, I'd like you to put in a proposal to the NIH." The proposal just barely fell short of the handful that the NIH was going to fund, mainly because they did not believe in Allen's hypothesis of the basis of Alzheimer's.

At that time I introduced him to philanthropist Joe Bryan in Greensboro. Mr. Bryan's wife, Kathleen Price Bryan, had suffered from Alzheimer's disease, and he took a great interest in trying to find a cause and cure for this devastating illness. Roses received a grant of $200,000 from Mr. Bryan to be able to lay the groundwork on which he could reapply to the NIH subsequently. This was effected, and Allen did a good job of staying in touch with Joe Bryan, keeping him informed about the progress of his research. When the time came to consider a new basic science facility

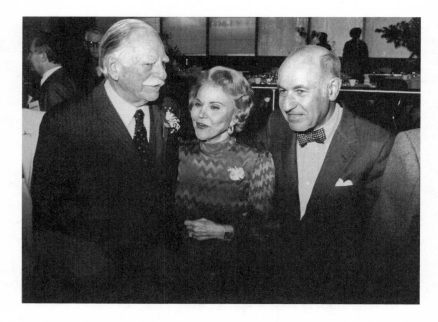

21   Dr. W. G. Anlyan with renowned friends: Mr. Joseph Bryan of Greensboro, N.C., a major benefactor of Duke University; and Ms. Eppie Lederer (Ann Landers), who visited Duke for numerous functions and dedications. 1990. DUMC Photography.

that would include the research program in Alzheimer's, it was logical to approach Joe Bryan for a $10 million gift for what amounted to a $28 million building. I made frequent visits to Joe Bryan, with and without Allen Roses. Subsequently Joe came forth with his $10 million gift and nailed down the facility. The rest of the money came from a variety of sources, including $10.75 million over several years from the hospital section of The Duke Endowment, $1.5 million from the Department of Radiology, $5 million from the Medical Center Building Fund, and $1.25 million from the Research Depreciation Fund.

We thought we were all set when we presented the plan to the Duke University Board of Trustees. For some reason, Ed Donnell, the former Montgomery Ward CEO, once again spoke up and said that the campus was being littered with ugly parking lots and that it was high time we did something about it. At that time, I said that we would build underground parking so that we would not be adding another visible parking lot. Early sample borings of the ground did not show any rock, and it seemed that we would be able to proceed with the underground parking without too much trouble or major cost. However, when the bulldozers came, there had to be extensive blasting through rock to create the deep hole for the building. The underground garage cost about two and a half times as much as an aboveground facility would have. Mr. Bryan came frequently from Greensboro, sometimes announced, sometimes unannounced, to follow the progress of the construction. It was almost like Cheops watching his pyramid go up at Giza on the outskirts of Cairo. He was very, very pleased, and Larry Nelson, the university and Medical Center architect, did an excellent job of keeping him informed as the building went up.

The assignment of space in this building brought to a head a long-standing tug-of-war between university and Medical Center. I had put together the whole lump sum for this building. And just as it was coming into the final phase of construction, Phillip Griffiths, the university provost, sent word that he would be in charge of assigning space in the building. I blew a gasket and said he absolutely would not—that the money from Mr. Bryan was given to the Medical Center, that the funds from The Duke Endowment were given from their hospital section, and that this was a Medical Center building and it was going to be assigned as such from the Medical Center. I even got The Duke Endowment to write a letter to that effect, so that the university administration at the time would back off, and they did. It had been a power play to get more control over the Medical Center, and we had resisted it.

IO

EVOLVING WITH THE UNIVERSITY

DUKE UNIVERSITY and the Duke Medical Center, comprising the Medical School and the hospital, are a single entity, a fact that has conferred many advantages on both parts of the system, as they developed in tandem. The relationship between the university and the Medical Center, however, has not always been an easy one. At times during my tenure the university administration tended to regard the Medical Center as a cash cow, to be milked for some of their objectives for which they did not have the funding. The administration could also at times make unilateral decisions that profoundly affected us. These tensions still occur between the university and the Medical Center. In general, such tensions can be healthy: they are inherent in the organism and inevitable as it changes and grows. They have been the subject of much debate and discussion— sometimes insufficient discussion—but the university machinery and the Medical Center continue to move forward, nonetheless.

Central to university–Medical Center tensions is the question of money. James Buchanan Duke left $10 million in a codicil to his will to create a medical school and hospital. But the entire capital project only took about $4 million, and the remaining $6 million—which, according to Dr. Davison, was mostly in Alcoa stock—was pooled with the university's endowment. The reason this was done, he told me, was that it was the middle of the Depression and he did not want to end up just having Alcoa stock, he wanted a more diversified investment base. So he and President Few agreed to put the $6 million into the general endowment of the university. I have not been able to verify Dr. Davison's story in any archival material either at the university or in The Duke Endowment, but it was clear that in the sixties the Medical School essentially had no endowment of its own, except for a $2 million contribution from the Ford Foundation. (The foundation had granted similar amounts to about twenty medical schools when it was formed, with the proviso that the schools never come back and ask the Ford Foundation for any more money, because it would not support medicine or health.) On June 30, 1989 (the year I left the Medical School to become chancellor of the university), the Medical Center—Medical School, Nursing School, and hospital—had built that initial $2 million endowment into one with a book value of $118,652,000. The market value was $146,937,000.

Back in the 1960s, after each of the annual budget sessions with the provost, I was left with the feeling that I was "stealing" from the undergraduate tuition collections to fund both the Medical School and the hospital. For the first few years of my tenure, the hospital operations were subsidized from the general pool of money from the university, as had been done traditionally since 1930. Then, when the university was struggling financially, I was asked by Barnes Woodhall (chancellor of the university), Marcus Hobbs (provost), and Chuck Huestis (vice president for business and finance)—the "troika" that was running the university in the interim between President Knight's resignation and President Sanford's appointment—whether I could forego the subsidy to the hospital for one year. I agreed to do that. Each year thereafter, when the matter came up, it was said that if I had been able to do without the hospital operational subsidy the year before, surely I could do it again. That was the end of the open-ended subsidy to hospital operations.

Not wanting to abandon completely the principle of some significant and regular support from the university, I raised the question of going back and looking at what that $6 million in Alcoa stock was worth in the late sixties, or as an alternative, to taking the last five years of subsidy that the hospital had received from the university budget and nailing that down as the Medical School share of the unassigned pool. The troika chose the latter. As it turned out, the five-year average of the unassigned income pool coming to the Medical School was at the level of 16 percent, so that percentage would continue indefinitely as the unassigned income pool rose. A small percentage, separate from the 16 percent for the Medical School, was also agreed upon for the School of Nursing and the Health Administration Program. In return for getting that fixed 16 percent contribution, I promised to pay the university for services that included the use of the road system, Duke Gardens, Duke Chapel, and security, and anything else that could be allocated. I persuaded the university leaders that medical students prayed only about 25 percent as much as other students, so we got a little bit of a break regarding the cost allocation of the Duke Chapel. But over the years, the 16 percent of unassigned income coming to the Medical Center had barely grown in dollar terms, whereas the expenses allocated to us had gone up and up. Quite often, the charges were increased without consultation. For example, all of a sudden the security force in the Medical Center was doubled, without anyone in our area having been asked whether we wanted it doubled or not. It may not have been a useless expense, but it certainly was imposed without any consultation.

When Nan Keohane became president of Duke University, she alluded to a "gauze curtain" that exists between the Medical Center and the university. I think that notion came about because of the Booz, Allen & Hamilton study that Barnes Woodhall had commissioned, which resulted in the university trustees setting aside a wedge of some eighty acres for the future development of the Medical Center. The university faculty interpreted the western border of that wedge as the gauze curtain that would keep the growing Medical Center from invading the university campus from that side. University anxieties were no doubt heightened by the unexpected speed with which the Medical Center developed its eighty-acre allotment.

At this point I had fallen into a trap made by our own success, because I now had to buy every parcel of land anywhere north of the Medical Center and Erwin Road, paying hard money that I had accrued, in order to have places for future expansion. Some of the land I bought at this time has since become part of the Durham Expressway, some has been used for the North Pavilion, the approximately 2,850-car Parking Garage II, and the 1,800-car Parking Garage III. We purchased all the land in the area as it became available, parcel by parcel. Also, we bought land on the other side of the Nearly New Shoppe, the medical wives' resale shop. Unfortunately, Duke President Sanford leased this land out to Metrosport Athletic Club without consulting me, and the only thing I got out of it was an honorary membership in that athletic club, which I have only used a handful of times in bad weather, substituting racquet ball for outdoor tennis. But that land was purchased by the Medical Center and should at some point be given back.

It has been my hope that the Levine Science Research Center, constructed in 1994, would assuage some of the anxieties of the university faculty, because it shows that all components of Duke University can work very well together, as they should. The Levine Building came about because for many decades interdisciplinary research in fields such as cell biology, molecular biology, and genetics programmatically combined the efforts of different components of the university, both in the arts and sciences and the Medical Center. For instance, genetics was a program run by botany, zoology, and the corresponding departments in the Medical Center. They applied together to the NIH and the NSF for funds for training programs, selected their trainees as a group, and met occasionally to discuss a variety of projects. The same with other areas, which at times included experimental psychology. Therefore, toward 1989, it became apparent that we might have the opportunity to bring under one roof all of the people who had traditionally worked in these university-wide programs, instead of just expanding separately in the Medical School basic sciences and on the university side within zoology, engineering, and botany. When I became chancellor of the university, I was assigned to pull it all together.

One of my early visits was to Charlotte to discuss with Leon Levine, the founder of Dollar Stores, the possibility of making a lead gift of $25 million toward a projected $70–75 million building. Mr. Levine and his family had been patients at Duke University Medical Center, and we were reasonably good friends. During one of the visits, Mr. Levine asked if he would contribute $10 million instead of $25 million, would I take it. I quickly said yes, subject to a final decision by the university administration and the trustees. We developed the funding on the basis of that lead gift, and we agreed to name the building for him. Dr. Charles Putman, the former chairman of radiology, who was then coordinating research grants in the university, was asked to oversee the further development of the building. This was fine with me, because I was never good at details. In the Medical Center, I had always left that level of work to Jane Elchlepp and Larry Nelson. My friendship with Leon Levine continued until he fell in arrears with his pledged contributions in the early years. Nan Keohane, who was Duke University president by then, asked me to go by and ask him to pay according to his written pledge. I was on my way to Washington and detoured by way of Charlotte to go and see him. I talked with him fairly firmly and apparently got him upset enough that he tracked me to Washington to tell me in an angry tone that he had never been talked to like that by anyone else. I pointed out that it was in his interest that I did that because it would not be useful to him for people to think of him as a person who did not deliver on his pledges. Subsequently, I stopped seeing Leon until the building was dedicated, and I believe we are probably back to being friends.

The Medical Center was always kept on a short leash when it came to financial support by the university, yet the growth of the university has been helped in no small measure by the generosity of grateful patients.

Among them was the businessman J. B. Fuqua. In the mid-sixties his wife, Dottie, called me to say he was dying of unknown causes at the Emory University Hospital. I had him flown up to Duke, where cardiologist Jim Morris took care of him, and within twenty hours they had diagnosed primary tuberculosis of the liver, a very, very rare disease. On antituberculous medication he got well. He was so grateful that he wanted to do something for Duke, and it turned out his principal interest was in creating a school of business. We had a foundering business school that was going nowhere. Mr. Fuqua put $10 million into it to get it overhauled, and it became the Fuqua School of Business. He has since invested considerably more in a variety of programs of the school, and much of the credit at the Duke end belongs to Tom Keller, dean of the Fuqua School. He served on Mr. Fuqua's board and has had a long-standing friendship with our benefactor. The Fuqua School is currently ranked in the top ten among its peers, according to annual surveys.

Then there was the Bryan family, who also were patients of the Medical Center. President Sanford told me one day that he thought he would like to ask Joe Bryan for $4 million for the construction of a student center on campus. My response to him was that he was the president and he should do what he wanted to do. Now Duke University students, faculty, and visitors can meet, eat, and enjoy art exhibits and theater as a community in the Bryan Center.

Dave Thomas, the founder of Wendy's, was one of Andy Wallace's grateful patients and a member of DUPAC (Duke University Preventive Approach to Cardiology), the cardiovascular rehabilitation program that Andy had founded. He gave money to establish the R. David Thomas Executive Conference Center at the Fuqua School of Business, which, incidentally, houses one of the best restaurants on campus.

At one point I had an inquiry from President Derek Bok of Harvard, asking how I had been so successful in attracting grateful patient money to help the non–Medical Center components of the university. The inquiry came through Elizabeth Dole, who had been a Duke trustee and was on the Board of Overseers at Harvard. I told her that Harvard would probably not be able to replicate what we had done, because the Harvard-affiliated teaching hospitals were separate corporations from the university, and I could not imagine the people at Mass General giving up their grateful

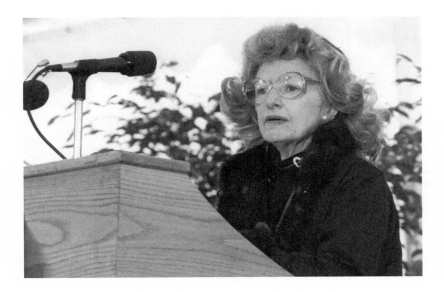

22 Mrs. Mary Duke Biddle Trent Semans, chair of The Duke Endowment and longtime trustee of Duke University, at the February 1986 groundbreaking ceremonies of the Joseph and Kathleen Bryan Research Building for Neurobiology. DUMC Photography.

patients to help something in Cambridge; I think Derek Bok found out that I was right.

Time and again, the steady evolution of the Medical Center and the university from a small southern institution into one with an international reputation has depended on the strength and commitment of particular individuals. Mary Duke Biddle Trent Semans and her husband, Jim Semans, are among the most notable figures in this story. Mary Semans is the granddaughter of Benjamin Newton Duke, a brother of James Buchanan Duke and a great benefactor of the university in his own right.

When I first came to Duke in 1949, Mary Semans was still Mary Trent; she had been widowed six months before, just before Christmas of 1948, when Joe Trent, a pioneering Duke thoracic surgeon, who was being trained to take over the chest surgery program, died of a lymphosarcoma at the age of about thirty-eight. Mary was understandably bereft, and we got to know each other slightly. Subsequently, John and Susan Dees introduced her to Jim Semans, a Hopkins-trained urologist who was practicing in Atlanta. A romance began, and they soon got married. Jim was offered a position on the faculty at Duke, and since that time they have worked together as a team in all of their numerous endeavors, including the N.C. School of the Arts in Winston-Salem, where Jim served as chairman of the board. (He also is chairman of the board of the Mary Duke Biddle Foundation, which was established by Mary Semans's mother.) They had three children together, to add to the four girls that Mary and Joe Trent had in earlier years.

Over the years, Mary became almost a sister to me, and I am sure she was a major factor in my appointment in 1990 as a trustee of The Duke Endowment, which she heads. In her capacity as a long-time Duke trustee and major benefactor, Mary was always very supportive of the evolution of the Medical Center. I don't know of a single instance when she opposed anything we proposed. Jim in his position was also very supportive, in his quiet way. After Jim's retirement, I provided him with an office in Baker House, and he became a member of the clinical investigation committee for research; he continues to serve in that capacity with great interest and devotion to this day.

Risk management and the whole process of preventing and dealing with litigation emerged during my tenure at the Medical Center. In this regard, the university and the Medical Center were both faced with the same problem, and we worked closely together in our response to it. In the early years of my administration, there was only one part-time legal counsel for the entire university—Ed Bryson, who was also a part-time professor at Duke Law School. Unfortunately, the world became much more litigious in the ensuing years. At first we could make do exclusively with an expanded university counsel's office, but in the seventies it became apparent that we needed a subset of lawyers within the Medical Center, and a staff for them, to deal with potential litigation. In the late 1980s we had a subset of university lawyers in the Medical Center and consultant legal counsels in Washington, New York City, Atlanta, and Durham. There were times when legal counsel would give me more than one option to choose from. Increasingly, however, I had to follow the advice given because I did not have the competence to arrive at an independent judgment.

I learned a lot about the law, since I had to be deposed for almost all of the hundreds of cases that occurred during my period. I might note that for every hour of deposition, you need at least an hour or two of preparation before being cross-examined by the litigants' lawyers. Although the number of lawsuits kept going up and up, it was impressive to see the prevention efforts instituted by the risk management component of the Medical Center law office. We needed lawyers specializing in personnel problems, and we had the firm of Fulbright & Jaworski advising us on potential litigation by employees and faculty; we had a separate firm in Atlanta advising us on tax issues and about the formal structure for the private diagnostic clinics in the seventies—they advised the doctors in the PDCs and interfaced with the Duke lawyers. Another set of lawyers on Wall Street was involved with the bonding issue for the North Division. I thought it ironic that the nation's experts in North Carolina bonds resided on Wall Street in New York City.

Personnel at the staff level would sometimes sue if they had been fired, and the unions were interested in maximizing the disaffection of biweekly employees who had been "mistreated" by the university. (Faculty and staff of Duke are paid monthly; employees in areas such as housekeeping are paid on a biweekly basis.) The faculty who took us to court generally were people we needed to fire for good cause. One example was an adjunct person on the open-heart team who was an alcoholic. We tried to fire him but had to settle by paying him a certain amount monthly (about $23,000 a year) because the university committee hearing the case was headed by a professor who couldn't understand why an alcoholic couldn't function on an open-heart team.

One of the constraints we had to deal with in my era was that the Medical Center had to conform to rules set by the university, which is not a 24-hour-a-day, 365-day-a-year operation with the kind of life-and-death responsibilities that we had to bear. We ran into the problem again in trying to change our length of pre-tenure service of faculty. The leadership of the Academic Council had no interest in having us lengthen the probationary period to eleven or twelve years from the university's standard seven years.

One piece of advice I received in my time was not to let the tail wag the dog, the tail being the Medical Center. I would point out that 60 percent of the faculty was in the Medical Center, and 75 percent of all people employed by the university were in the Medical Center. That remark did not win me any friends.

When President Sanford was about to retire, he asked me what my greatest fear was for the future of the Medical Center. I told him that my greatest fear was external to the Medical Center: it was that the university would become a vestigial appendix of the Medical Center, and no medical center today can be among the top five in the country if it is appended to a vestigial university. My concern, therefore, was to see the university continue to strive for even higher quality, quality that was strong and enduring. This concern lay behind my constant efforts to break through the gauze curtain and build joint programs and research buildings where university and Medical School faculty and students could work side by side. Fortunately, the university has been led by people who have pursued excellence in hiring and who have supported the academic programs by investing in infrastructure, just as we did in the Medical Center. The result has been gratifying, with the university as a whole rising in the national rankings and the Medical Center continuing to be held in high regard. When I left the Medical Center in 1989 to become chancellor of the university, we were ranked number 3 by *U.S. News and World Report*. I was immensely pleased that it was ranked number 3 again in 2001.

The very last thing I did in the Medical Center was, after much thought, to eliminate smoking. Up to 1988 no medical centers in this area had banned smoking; I don't know if they had them in other parts of the country. I thought it was ridiculous for us to allow active or passive smoke inhalation in the Medical Center when we were trying to do so much to prevent or cure disease before people got inoperable cancer of the lung. With the support of the Medical School advisory committee (MedSAC), made up of all the chairmen, we also passed a rule that smoking would not be allowed in private offices. There were two reasons for this decision: first, permitting smoking in private offices would be discriminatory to lower-level employees who did not have a private office in which to hide; second, the air-conditioning systems spread smoke throughout the Medical Center. We decided that the only place where smoking would be allowed would be outdoors. Now we have complaints by people saying that to get into the Medical Center they have to go through a cloud of smoke and piles of cigarette butts, and the current Medical Center administration is faced with trying to do something about that.

I got surprisingly little flak about the pending no-smoking rule, even though a few of the people in the top administration were smokers. One person objected on the basis that James Buchanan Duke had made his money from tobacco, and here I was banning smoking; I pointed out that he didn't make his big money from tobacco, but from hydroelectric power and the aluminum business. He got out of the tobacco business when the Sherman Anti-Trust Act was passed, because he felt that tobacco would no longer be a source of wealth. One subsequent objector said, "How can you ban tobacco when Mr. Duke's statue in front of Duke Chapel is with a cigar in his hand?" I pointed out that he was outdoors.

II

BUILDING LINKS TO THE
COMMUNITY IN DURHAM
AND BEYOND

W HEN I GRADUATED in 1949, I was very familiar with the town-gown friction that existed in New Haven. It was essentially the irritation that a less-than-affluent community, the "town," feels for the casually careless disdain and wealth of an academic community, the "gown."

In New Haven, there was a strictly two-party interface of town and gown, although the town was multilayered, with a variety of subsets of population. (New England Yankees were at the top of the social list, and going down from them there was the large Italian colony, the Jewish colony, and the black population.) Yale dealt mainly with the mayor rather than the townspeople themselves. In the late forties the university did nothing visible to enhance the community, such as paying taxes or mounting joint ventures. I understand from what I have read recently that under its current president, Rick Levin, there are many common ventures and some taxes are paid.

The principal difference between Yale and Duke while I was at the Medical Center was that there were three distinct communities in Durham, making for a three-way interface—the university, the white inhabitants of Durham (many of whom had strong affiliation to the University of North Carolina in Chapel Hill and/or Watts Hospital in Durham), and Durham's black population, including its black physicians.

In Durham, the interface problem with Watts Hospital and its physicians got transferred to the Durham County Hospital, subsequently called Durham Regional Hospital, although an increasing number of Duke-trained residents started to practice in the community. For the most part, community physicians did not have admitting privileges at Duke but were given courtesy appointments to come to any conferences they wished. One of the few services where there seemed to be a little more harmony was orthopedics, largely thanks to the efforts of Dr. Lenox Baker and his successor, Dr. Leonard Goldner, who saw to it that the orthopedic surgeons in the community were much more visible on teaching rounds and in conferences. However, in medicine and surgery for the most part the relationships were much more distant. Clearly, the leading surgeon in the community was James Davis, and he was an alumnus and strong supporter of the medical school at UNC–Chapel Hill. For a while, when Duke's new affiliation with Durham Regional Hospital was being considered, there was a definite consideration whether the community hospital's affiliation should be with the residency program at Chapel Hill rather than at Duke. Duke won out, so several of our residency programs have rotations through Durham's community hospital.

In terms of our interface with the black leadership, we did not have a black full-time appointee on the staff of Duke Medical Center until Dr. Stead appointed endocrinologist Charles Johnson in 1970 as a full-time faculty member of the medical PDC. This was a somewhat difficult transition for Dr. Johnson, and I spent many hours listening to some of the problems he encountered. Subsequently, Dr. Onye Akwari was appointed to the surgical staff, and there started to be sort of a relationship whereby Dr. Johnson and Dr. Akwari would refer patients to each other. The problem disappeared for the most part, in my view, as we recruited more and more minority students and residents and eventually senior staff. With the dissolution of the all-black Lincoln Hospital, all the black physicians in the community had admitting privileges to Durham County Hospital and it ceased to be a problem.

We have a good relationship that evolved over many years with the Lincoln Community Clinic, which principally serves Durham's African American community, and which is under the leadership of Dr. Evelyn Schmidt, a pediatrician trained at Duke and one of my former students. She was selected by a committee headed by Dr. Charles Watts, the renowned African American surgeon in the Durham community, despite the fact that she is white and originally came from the New York area. She has been very well accepted by the black community as well as by Duke physicians. It may be that pediatricians are easier to get along with than, say, surgeons. Her success was facilitated by having supporters of Dr. Schmidt such as Dr. Sam

Katz, the chairman of pediatrics and a far-sighted leader in the field of children's health, involved throughout the evolution of these relationships.

Dr. Charles Watts is one of Durham's most eminent citizens. A graduate of Morehouse College in Atlanta, he went to Howard University School of Medicine and trained there in surgery. After his surgical training, he looked for a suitable place to practice where he would have full privileges. He chose Durham's black Lincoln Hospital, knowing full well that he would not have admitting privileges at Watts Hospital (as Durham's community hospital was then called), which was not integrated, nor at Duke, where we had a full-time staff. Dr. Watts eventually got a courtesy appointment from Dr. Hart, so that he could attend all the conferences and rounds. In the early fifties, the backlog for admissions to the only black surgical Nott Ward at Duke Hospital became so long that Dr. Hart established a satellite service under one of the younger faculty, Dr. Shingleton, at Lincoln Hospital. In 1952 I spent six months on that rotation and most of my operating experience was there that year. On one occasion, Dr. Shingleton, who was to supervise me on a particular operation, was delayed, and I can recall Dr. Watts coming in and saying, "Why don't you proceed, and I'll keep an eye on you?" For that, I have been eternally grateful.

I am still embarrassed by an incident that took place during my internship year. I went to the Center Theater in downtown Durham to see a movie with my family, and Dr. Watts and his wife were standing in a separate line leading to the balcony for "colored" people. I have never been able to obliterate that memory.

My background in Egypt had given me a variety of relationships with people of color. The Egyptians themselves—people of Arab descent, and not Coptic—for the most part are brown-skinned, not black. The only blacks in Egypt were the Sudanese or came from Nubia, which is tucked between the Sudan and southern Egypt. In general, they were servants in Egypt. There was no one in the governmental or social hierarchy who was black. I think my biggest shock when coming to the United States was seeing my first American black. I immediately thought of speaking Arabic to him until I realized I was in a different country and that blacks here did not speak that language.

I don't think this early experience of blacks in Egypt affected my relationships with black patients in any way or my relationships with other people. It was somewhat distressing to see that there were always two water fountains and two bathrooms, and that this division even went so far as the morgue at Duke Hospital, which came with four subcomponents, differentiating sex and color. The same was true in the blood bank, where there was a separate, recognizable stamp to mark blood that had come from black donors (which I always ignored). Segregation remained in force until 1963. At that time, Deryl Hart was president of Duke University and Taylor Cole was provost, and they persuaded the Duke University Board of Trustees to do away with the racial barrier for students, patients, and everyone else. Finally and officially, the whole segregation business went out the window, and we were able to have one communal water fountain and the "colored" labels on the bathrooms were removed.

Shortly after that happened, I helped recruit Bernard Amos, an Australian educated in England, as a tissue immunologist. He was looking for laboratory space, and he persuaded me in 1964 that we would never, even with an epidemic, use all the bathrooms we had. And so we converted some of the bathrooms in the newer buildings to laboratory space.

In those days, our involvement with the community was to take care of anyone who showed up at our doors. We have consistently taken care of more poor citizens of Durham County than all of the other public and state-supported hospitals of North and South Carolina, according to Duke Endowment statistics. We did not really have much "community involvement" as such, except piecemeal, such as the collaboration by the Department of Pediatrics with Evelyn Schmidt and the Lincoln Community Center. Many other efforts were random or sporadic.

When I became chancellor of the university, I was very interested in getting Duke involved with the school system, but we did not get any support at the top and the efforts did not get anywhere. The situation is different today, however. After having assumed the responsibility for Durham Regional Hospital and with it the subsidiary Lincoln Community Center, Duke has the only hospital system in the whole community. Therefore, in his wisdom, Dr. Snyderman recruited Dr. Jean Spaulding from her private practice in the Durham community to spearhead any other bridge-building efforts that the Medical Center should undertake. She has accomplished these community efforts with great sensitivity and effectiveness.

From the vantage point of the work I am currently doing with the Durham community, I realize that there are a lot of issues that I did not fully appreciate earlier. For example, I realize one group we probably should have identified more aggressively is the practicing doctors in the community. Some of them, of course, had joint appointments on the Duke faculty, but many did not, and they need to be handled with care and diplomacy.

Their support is critical to having some unity in caring for the community. Our referring physicians in the town of Durham and beyond remain an important constituency, since the patients they refer to us are crucial to the survival of the hospital. It is interesting that even our own graduates regard themselves to some degree as competitors of Duke: the closer they are to Durham, the more competitive they tend to be; the further away they are, the more relaxed they will be about referring patients to Duke.

The university's involvement with medical care delivery beyond the Duke Medical Center has not always been successful. Accepting Sea Level Hospital as a gift to Duke University was a terrible mistake. It happened in the course of Duke's first major fundraising drive under Duke President Doug Knight, when the university got a four-to-one matching grant from the Ford Foundation. Any gift received under that program that could be matched was welcomed by Doug's fundraising crew, which consisted initially of Everett Hopkins and Frank Ashmore who joined the university development staff after Doug's appointment. So when the opportunity presented itself in 1969 to receive as a gift the entire eighty-bed Sea Level Hospital and about two thousand acres of land nearby, the university—in consultation with Dr. Woodhall—was quick to accept, because it qualified for the Ford Foundation match.

Sea Level Hospital is located in Carteret County, near Beaufort and Morehead City, on the eastern shore of North Carolina. The hospital was created by Dan Taylor and his family (the gift was made by the Taylor Foundation, whose members were Dan Taylor, his brothers, William and Leslie, and their father, Maltby). The Taylors were natives of Sea Level, and I guess they felt guilty about moving to Palm Beach and Norfolk and abandoning their native turf, so they built a hospital for the people still abiding in their old home hamlet. There was no reason ever to put a hospital in that location, when people could be hospitalized in Morehead City, a drive of thirty to forty-five minutes away. Sea Level was an utter millstone around my neck, and as soon as I could delegate the day-to-day supervision to Harvey Estes, chairman of the Department of Community and Family Medicine, I did so. I still had to go once a year, usually in the duck-hunting season, to visit the facility. We were always put up at the Sea Level Inn, and on most occasions they put me in Mr. Taylor's private suite, which was very elaborate, unlike most other parts of the Inn.

There had been five doctors in Sea Level when the gift was accepted by Duke, so it appeared to be safe as far as the doctor population was concerned, which in turn indicated that the hospital population would remain at an acceptable level. However, Dr. Peacock, the surgeon who was the mainstay, died shortly after we took over the hospital, and soon we were down to two doctors, one of whom was on drugs and the other an alcoholic. We spent the next decade or more trying to recruit physicians to Sea Level so as to keep the beds full. It was a mess, because very few physicians would want to raise a family in that area, since there were no schools and no professional equals closer than Beaufort and Morehead City, thirty-five miles away. Eventually we solved the problem by turning some of the beds into a nursing home facility and retaining only a small number of acute-care beds.

In 1974 we even enticed Sailors' Snug Harbor, a privately endowed retirement home for "old, worn-out sailors" that had been located on Staten Island, New York, since its founding in the early nineteenth century to move down to Sea Level. (The home's original charter had been drawn up by Alexander Hamilton.) The administration of Sailors' Snug Harbor were not particularly happy with Staten Island, and they were looking for a new location. Since they owned a lot of real estate under Washington Square, in Manhattan, they were well endowed. We brought them down to visit Sea Level, and we wined and dined them and told them how great it would be for retired sailors to spend their last years on the edge of the water. All the time, we were thinking that this would fill up the hospital with older people when they got sick. When they moved to Sea Level, they brought their own ambulatory care system with them, and except for the part-time use of one of the physicians who practiced at Sea Level Hospital, their people never occupied more than one or two beds.

In the early seventies I also tried to get the people who ran the Carolina Caribbean Corporation, which was responsible for developing Hound Ears, outside of Boone, to create a retirement complex on the two thousand acres of land that was part of the gift, so that we could increase the population of Sea Level—again, to provide more potential patients for the hospital. Unfortunately, about this time, the corporation went broke. I tried to get other developers to come and look at the land, suggesting that this might be the next Hilton Head, the popular resort north of Charleston, South Carolina. On one occasion I chartered a plane to fly a group from New York over the property and the surrounding area to survey it from the air. Because this was a restricted area, I had received permission from the commanding general at Cherry Point, the Marine base, to fly over. Cedar

Island, which is in juxtaposition to Sea Level, was used for target practice by fighter planes, and somehow we got our signals crossed, because as we were flying at a relatively low altitude over the Sea Level property, planes dropping bombs came to meet us. The New York developers went home as soon as possible.

I also well remember one of my annual visits to Sea Level, always very social occasions. I excused myself and went to bed around nine, while the reveling went on. At dawn, I found myself in a duck blind seated between one man holding an ancient blunderbuss, which he had never fired, and another gentleman holding a bottle of Courvoisier. The ducks had nothing to fear from them. I couldn't say the same for myself.

We developed an affiliated clinic with nearby Harker's Island, and we would send the physicians from Sea Level there to see if there were any candidates for hospitalization. All of this time I would go back to the trustees of The Duke Endowment, promising them there would be light at the end of the tunnel and hoping they would continue to support in a small way the operations of this misbegotten gift. The eventual solution was to give Sea Level Hospital to the Morehead City hospital to run as they saw fit.

Highland Hospital in Asheville, in the mountains of North Carolina, presented somewhat similar problems—those of trying to run and make profitable a facility far removed from the Medical Center. Highland Hospital is the 125-bed private psychiatric facility whose main claim to fame is that Zelda Fitzgerald, F. Scott Fitzgerald's wife, perished there in a tragic fire in 1948. The facility was given to Duke University in 1939, after twenty-five years of "successful operation," by its founder, Dr. Robert S. Carroll. It functioned originally under the jurisdiction of the university. The university comptroller, a man named Alfred Smith Brower, had his own apartment in Highland Hospital, and he did not want the Medical Center to play a role of any significance.

From 1940 to 1951 the Department of Psychiatry at Duke was very weak. In 1953, when Dr. Ewald Busse became chairman, things began to change, and Highland was fully integrated into the Medical Center in 1967 as a division of the Department of Psychiatry. The psychiatrists, psychologists, and social workers at Highland held academic appointments in the department. For many years, the hospital represented a valuable resource for the area, and its staff did a good job of teaching as well as providing clinical care. However, quality control from a distance of more than two hundred miles was always a problem. In addition, Duke's lawyers discovered that

Highland presented a potential danger to our tax-exempt status if it was not used sufficiently for teaching—and the teaching level was at times hard to maintain.

Though Highland Hospital had potential as an excellent facility, it became an ever-greater drain on the finances and the managerial capacity of the Department of Psychiatry, and finally, when Keith Brodie—himself a psychiatrist—was president of Duke University, it was sold.

12

THE CHANGING NATIONAL SCENE

THE CHANGES THAT were taking place in the Duke Medical Center's structure and programs did not, of course, occur in a vacuum. All around it, in the United States and abroad, things were in flux: medical training, surgical and diagnostic techniques, medicines and treatments, and the delivery of care were all transforming in the light of new science, new laws and social programs, and changes in the economy. The Duke Medical Center was a leader in many areas and learned and adapted the innovations of others. Associated institutions such as professional and scientific societies were also adapting to the times; they too were often in the forefront of change.

Part and parcel of my work of directing and developing the Duke Medical Center was to be active on this vital national scene. I participated, for example, in the work of the Association of American Medical Colleges (AAMC) in a variety of posts. The association was organized in 1890 to represent the medical schools of the United States. However, it did not have much power or authority; it had been regarded as a "deans' chowder society" until it was reorganized in the late 1960s, when John Parks, dean of George Washington Medical School, was president. Dr. Parks asked me to head the reorganization committee—named the "ways and means committee"—and our recommendations included increasing the dues sevenfold, as well as creating a Council of Deans, a Council of Academic Societies, and a Council of Teaching Hospitals. In 1968 I was asked to be the first chair of the Council of Deans. From 1970 to 1971 I served as chairman of the Assembly, which represented all three councils. After the student Viet-

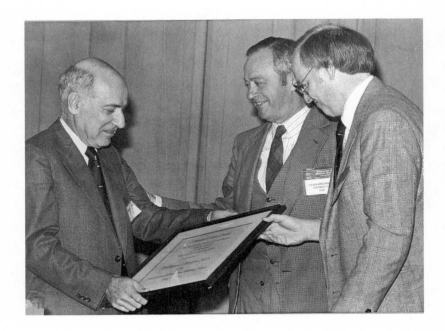

23   Dr. W. G. Anlyan receiving the Abraham Flexner Award for Service to Medical Education at the AAMC Convention of Washington, D.C., October 28, 1980. Dr. Julius Krevans, chancellor of the University of California, San Francisco, and Dr. John Gronvall, dean of the University of Michigan School of Medicine made the presentations. From personal archive of author.

nam demonstrations, we created an Organization of Student Representatives to give medical students a forum within the AAMC. I served on the task force on physician supply from 1987 to 1989 and have been a member of the AAMC/AHA (American Hospital Association) liaison committee on medical education since 1971.

By 1970 I had also started attending the informal meetings of the vice presidents' group, the Association of Academic Health Centers (AAHC). It was about this time that I was given the title of vice president for health affairs at Duke, so in some sense it became part of my responsibilities to attend these meetings. I found that the organization was operated by one low-level executive director and a secretary, and essentially run out of the pocket of whoever was president for a two-year term. At that time it was Randy Batson, a pediatrician who had been the dean at Vanderbilt. Shortly after I joined, they asked me to be on the governing council, and I felt that that organization needed to become more formally organized. They elected me president in 1973, and I served as president in 1974–75.

I tried to bring the organization into a more formal group by having them become part of the AAMC. The AAHC deals primarily with the problems intrinsic to academic medical centers, representing all the health professions schools. The AAMC has a much stronger program in lobbying and dealing with Congress and the public, so they fulfilled complementary functions and represented the medical schools, teaching hospitals, and medical faculty organizations.

John Cooper was head of the AAMC at that time, and he was against any union with the AAHC. He did not want any competition from the vice presidents' group. Subsequently in its history, the AAHC recruited John Hogness, who had been the founding president of the Institute of Medicine of the National Academy of Sciences. Thereafter he was president of the University of Washington at Seattle. He came back to Washington as the full-time president of the AAHC. Unfortunately, there was an old rivalry between John Hogness and John Cooper, so I was never able to get a rapprochement. (I have often wondered if the sibling rivalry between Cooper and Hogness emanated from the fact that I was the emissary of the search committee for the newly created presidency of the AAMC in the 1960s and had offered the position initially to John Hogness; Cooper may have learned of this. The search committee included the then head of the AAMC, Bob Glaser, and Bob Howard, who was dean of the medical school at the University of Minnesota and who was elected head of the AAMC the following year. Until recently, I thought that the three of us on the committee had been able to keep the priority a secret.) On Cooper's retirement in the late eighties, I gave it one more try to bring the associations together, but that failed as well, and they maintained their separate identities. There seems, after all, to be a spot in the sun for both organizations to function separately. Roger Bulger succeeded John Hogness at the AAHC, and Bulger has done an outstanding job and become a real statesman.

The leadership at Duke has had a long relationship with the National Library of Medicine. Wilburt Davison was a member of its board when it was still the Armed Forces Library. Subsequently named the National Library of Medicine, today this is the biomedical information resource of the nation and, in fact, the leader in the world. It has led in the evolution of computer and information technology availability for every health institution in this country. It is a magnificent jewel in the crown of the National

Institutes of Health, and, for a relatively small amount of money, it does a great deal of good.

In the late sixties Barnes Woodhall was a member of the Board of Regents of the library and, in his final year of service, he became chairman of that board. I was invited to join the board after Dr. Woodhall finished his term, and I became board chairman in 1971–72. Since 1988 I have been a member of the board of the Friends of the National Library of Medicine and on its executive committee since 1991.

In the meantime, I had also become founding chairman of the board of EDUCOM (Education Communications), a position I held from 1963 to 1968. This group grew out of a 1963 AAMC deans' meeting at the airport Hilton in Atlanta. (The AAMC always seemed to meet at inexpensive airport hotels to keep costs down.) One of the most inspiring talks I ever heard at AAMC was given by Dr. James Grier Miller, a brilliant individual and a professor of psychiatry at the University of Michigan, on the future of the information sciences in education, with a broad focus on their impact on universities.

Following Miller's presentation and after dinner, Jim Miller, Gene Stead, and I got together, and we talked about how wonderful it would be to establish an interuniversity information network. I was asked to be founding chairman, with Jim Miller as the principal scientist and the brains behind it. To get the organization started, I helped recruit the chief financial officer of the University of Pittsburgh, Edison Montgomery, as the first full-time president. Over the years, it changed from being a broad academic enterprise to being more focused on computer scientists and the information sciences and to sharing resources on a national basis. EDUCOM is now a big interuniversity network with headquarters in Princeton, mainly because one of the succeeding presidents lived there.

In 1973, two years after I had finished my term as chairman of the Assembly of the AAMC, I became chairman of a newly created national body called the Coordinating Council on Medical Education (CCME). The five "parents" of the CCME were the AAMC, the American Medical Association, the American Board of Medical Specialties, the Council of Medical Specialty Societies, and the American Hospital Association. Our Chicago sessions unfortunately resembled those of the United Nations Security Council: the charter of the CCME provided that if one organization vetoed a proposal, the whole issue died. So for three or four years, I would come back from these meetings wondering what in heck was going on and why these five organizations could not agree on any important decisions in medical edu-

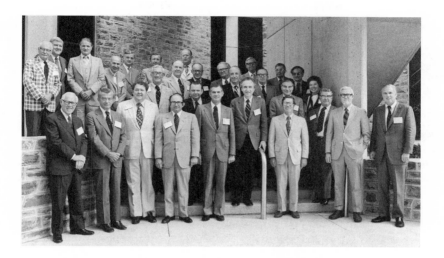

24 National leaders at the first Private Sector Conference, September 21, 1977. The conference was on the national challenges affecting medicine and provided a venue for leaders in the medical field to get to know each other better in smaller settings. DUMC Photography.

cation, especially at a time when the private sector—which we all represented—had to interact more and more with the federal government.

This was very much on my mind when, in July 1976, the bicentennial year of the founding of our country, I sat down and wrote an editorial for *Perspectives*, Duke's medical alumni magazine. The column took the form of a letter from me to Benjamin Rush, one of our founding fathers and, I believe, the only physician to sign the Declaration of Independence. It was a dialogue between Rush, who was in heaven, and me, at my summer home in Beech Mountain. It talked about some of the things that we couldn't seem to solve in the United States any more. It was a light way to approach some serious problems. Alex McMahon, who had just become chairman of the Board of Trustees of Duke University, wrote me a note asking me what I was going to do about it. That is how the Private Sector Conferences at Duke came about.

One of the primary purposes of the conferences was to unify the nongovernmental components of health care in the country, namely the private sector, including the five major associations. While we were facing a variety of external issues that nibbled at our independence (increased government funding of health care brought with it ever increasing conditions placed on the way we operated), we were threatened as well with being torn asunder by internal forces. Unless the private sector stood together, we would be picked off one by one.

So in 1977 I invited thirty to thirty-five of the top leaders in the country, including representatives of the five warring organizations, to Duke to discuss "The Future of the Private Sector in Medical Care." In subsequent years, conferences focused on broad issues such as "The Private Sector and Cost Containment," "Financing Health Care" (and what that implied for teaching, research and teaching hospitals), "Can the Private Sector Lead the Evolution of Medicine in the 1980s?," and "The Financial Support of Health Care of the Elderly and Indigent" (Joseph Califano, secretary of health, education and welfare, attended that one). Attendees included medical providers and educators, representatives of corporations and foundations, and influential members of government and of professional publications. It was a broad selection of people with special expertise and particular points of view. The idea was to let them get to know each other without any rigid agenda, so that they might get to respect and trust one another.

Three of the principal adversaries at that time—and three of the main attendees—were John Cooper, Jim Sammons, and David Rogers. John Cooper of the AAMC didn't really trust Jim Sammons of the American Medical Association. The AMA was big and powerful, the AAMC was a fledgling deans' club, and the leaders of the two rarely got together. When I became chairman of the AAMC's Council of Deans and helped recruit John Cooper from his position as dean of science at Northwestern University to the presidency of the AAMC, I made every effort to encourage him to meet with the executive vice president of the AMA to see if they could collaborate more effectively. Both Cooper and Sammons were fairly flamboyant, hard-nosed characters. Sammons might be regarded as ultraconservative; he stood as the champion of all practicing physicians, and some of his detractors referred to him as being to the right of Attila the Hun. Cooper was a little more progressive, slightly more liberal, but still quite a dictator in his own bailiwick. The third person involved in this power struggle within the medical establishment was David Rogers, president of the Robert Wood Johnson Foundation. Ideologically, David was a fairly liberal individual; he espoused the usual do-everything-for-everybody approach. In other words, Sammons and Cooper were for minimum governmental intrusion into the lives of people, and Rogers was the great social do-gooder taking care of the poor and the needy.

I am happy to say that at the end of the first Private Sector Conference, Sammons, Rogers and Cooper seemed to understand each other and get along, and subsequently there were no great problems in getting them all to think together at Private Sector Conferences. Duke University Medical Center continues to host the annual conferences.

Incidentally, David Rogers was indirectly involved in one of the two major job offers I received during my years at the Medical Center. Rogers had been chairman of medicine at Vanderbilt, and subsequently became dean of the Johns Hopkins medical school. It was fairly well known that he was having a rugged time with the faculty there. When Gustav Lienhard was board chairman of the newly formed Robert Wood Johnson Foundation, in 1971 or 1972, he called me up one day and asked to visit me for a couple of hours. He wouldn't tell me what it was about. When he arrived, he asked me if I would like to be considered for the presidency of the Robert Wood Johnson Foundation. I pointed out to him that I had a lot of good things going at Duke and that it was a bad time for me to consider such a generous offer; also I could not really see myself going to a desk job outside an academic medical center and getting my kicks out of shuffling papers. As we were saying good-bye, he asked me if I knew any deans he should consider. I told him about Rogers, who was not happy at Hopkins. Rogers subsequently became the new president of the new Robert Wood Johnson Foundation.

My other major job offer came from President Bart Giamatti of Yale when he was looking for a new dean for Yale Medical School. I had gotten to know Giamatti from alumni meetings, and I liked him immensely. He called me one day and asked, "Bill, what would it take to bring you back home?" I thought about the cold winters in New Haven and the fact that I had recruited a great many superb people to Duke and was having fun doing what I was doing. I begged off politely from that possibility as well. I know I made the right decision because I have watched closely some of the misery the deans have gone through at Yale, particularly because the New Haven Hospital, or the Yale–New Haven Hospital, as it is now known, is not under the control of the head of the medical school. In fact, until I became a member of the President's Council at Yale and chairman of the medical center subcomponent, the dean at Yale was not even on the board of the hospital; I insisted that Yale's president, Benno Schmidt, make the medical dean a member. I always thanked the Lord that our Duke Hospital was under the same corporate umbrella as the Medical School, under the same chancellor, and under one set of trustees of the university. However, it should be added that nowadays owning a hospital might be viewed by university presidents as a major liability.

Jack Whitehead, a former patient at Duke who at one point had considered putting his Whitehead Institute for Biomedical Research at Duke (it went to MIT), was concerned that when the era of Mary Lasker and her group had passed, it would leave a void in the public debate influencing health-related legislation, particularly as it concerns research support, in Washington. (Mary Lasker was a well-connected private citizen with a deep interest in medical research who had several powerful friends on congressional committees overseeing such legislation.) Whitehead founded Research!America in 1989, and was able to get former Connecticut senator Lowell Weicker, who had been a champion of the NIH, as the full-time president of the new organization, headquartered in Alexandria, Virginia. Jack asked me to be on the board.

Research!America is a not-for-profit public education and advocacy group based in Alexandria, Virginia. Its work is supported by the roughly four hundred member organizations, including academic institutions and teaching hospitals, research institutes, professional and scientific societies, businesses and foundations, trade associations, and health organizations.

Unfortunately, Senator Weicker, who had insisted at the beginning that he was through with politics, saw the opportunity of running for the governorship of Connecticut. This led to a period of well over a year of indecision, with nothing moving until Weicker made up his mind. When he finally decided to run for governor, Jack Whitehead recruited Mary Woolley, who has been president of Research!America ever since.

When Jack Whitehead died unexpectedly in 1992, some members of the Research!America board suggested that I become the new chairman of the board. I served in that capacity for four years. I felt that the first order of business was to build a decent launching pad, because Jack had run a rather helter-skelter organization. There were no set dates for future meetings; they usually came about at the last minute, when Jack had a clear spot on his schedule. There was no formal organization, nor were there by-laws. My objective was to stabilize and organize the group, with an executive committee and a broader board, all of whom would be participants in the affairs of the organization. In the course of my third year as chairman, it

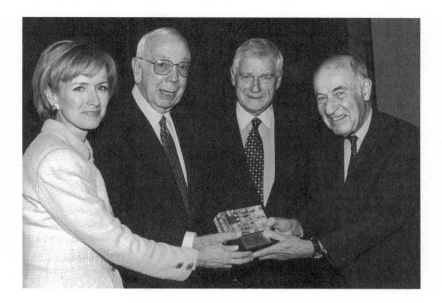

25   Dr. W. G. Anlyan receiving the first annual award for Lifetime Achievement as
an Advocate for Medical Research from Research!America in Washington, D.C., at
the National Academy of Science, March 1977. (L–R) Judy Woodruff of CNN and
former Duke Trustee, who presented the award; former congressman Paul Rogers,
who succeeded Dr. Anlyan as chairman of the board of Research!America; and
Senator Mark O. Hatfield, who for many years had championed biomedical research
in Congress. From personal archive of author.

became apparent that I had accomplished my limited goal, so I indicated
to the board that I would not seek renewal of the chairmanship after the
fourth year. I appointed Ike Robinson, the former head of Duke Hospital
who was then vice chancellor for health affairs at Vanderbilt, as chairman
of the search committee to identify the next chairman, and he very fortunately came back suggesting former congressman Paul Rogers who served
on many nonprofit boards as a senior partner of the prestigious Hogan &
Hartson law firm in Washington. Paul will be completing his sixth year as
chair in 2002.

   Paul Rogers and Mary Woolley have done an outstanding job in building up the board membership and the membership as a whole so that Research!America has become a major force in the promotion—to the public

and in Congress—of biomedical research. The goal to double the NIH budget now appears to be attainable with strong bipartisan support. I am still a member of the executive committee and the board, and attend most of the meetings, which are most often in Washington.

As I think about the work done by Research!America, and the way we go about doing it, I find that nothing in modern communications technology really supplants the interpersonal transactions that take place throughout the biomedical world. Modern technology is additive and perhaps speeds up and improves communication, but interpersonal knowledge and relationships continue to be very important. The younger generation in Washington is every bit as aware of the importance of interpersonal relationships as we were in my day.

My involvement with the world outside Duke was not restricted to nonprofit medical and research organizations. I also had a wonderful experience serving on the board of directors of G. D. Searle and Company, and subsequently Monsanto, from 1974 to 1991. The connection began in 1973 when I was recruited by Dan and Bill Searle, and their brother-in-law, Wes Dixon, to join the board of Searle, which was then developing from a one-product, medium-sized company into a major pharmaceutical firm with many products. At the time Dan was chairman of the board, Bill was vice chairman, and Wes was president, and the board met monthly in the Chicago area.

By 1976 it had become apparent that the Searles were ready to give up the day-to-day leadership of their board and their company. The year 1977 saw Jimmy Carter become president, and in the changeover of administrations, Donald Rumsfeld became available for a new chapter in his life. Rumsfeld had been chief of staff to President Ford and a former secretary of defense; he was also an old friend of the Searle family and in earlier years the congressman from that area. The Searles and Dixon, seeing their opportunity, came to visit me to get my concurrence in offering the position of Searle CEO to Rumsfeld.

One of the most impressive things about the Searle board was that I was one of just two physicians on the board; the others were all no-nonsense hard-nosed businessmen, most of them from the Chicago area. There were about ten meetings a year; they started at nine and finished at noon, and the board went through the business at hand in a very brisk way. Initially, there were no women and no African Americans on the board, but eventually a woman was appointed who was in the publishing business in New York and an African American man who was the head of his own food company

in Chicago. Almost everyone in the room smoked pipes or cigars or ciga-
rettes, and I didn't see how the woman, who didn't smoke, could survive;
she must have been used to boardrooms filled with smoke.

In or about 1985 Don Rumsfeld helped sell G. D. Searle and Company
to Monsanto. On the recommendation of Rumsfeld, I was the only member of the Searle board who was asked to continue on the subsidiary board
with Monsanto. The styles of operation were very different as the leadership changed, and I learned something about management, both good and
bad, from each one. The Searle family ran the company as a family affair.
Old Jack Searle, the father, sat in the meetings in my initial years. He was a
grumpy soul with an angry face because he wasn't happy with the way his
sons were running the company, but he never said a word except "hello"
and "good-bye." Dan and Bill Searle and Wes Dixon ran the company like
a family team, and everything was very congenial, polite, and proper. Don
Rumsfeld, by contrast, ran it like a tough businessman, with very little
sense of humor; things tended to be cut and dried. He did assemble a good
team with his chief operating officer, John Robson, who had been the administrator for the Civil Aeronautics Board (it was he who deregulated
the airlines, even though Kahn, who came in under the Carter administration, took all the credit). Robson had much more of a sense of humor
and was more fun to be with at dinner than Rumsfeld. Don Rumsfeld, like
Dan Searle before him, tended to be on several other boards, especially
around Chicago. One of the things that bothered me when I was on the
compensation committee was that it seemed that the members were com-
paring salaries of the boards they were all on and used that information as
a tool to jack one another's compensation up. I guess that's the way business runs.

Both organizations covered a lot of territory in the meetings. In contrast
to Dan Searle, who was a somewhat quiet, nervous person at stockholder
meetings, Rumsfeld was like a lion tamer walking into the cage. He was
well-prepped, much as a secretary of defense would be at a news conference.
Under Dan Searle, the Searle stock had taken a slight dive from fourteen
to eleven dollars; when Rumsfeld took over, with John Robson's help he
managed to get a few new drugs that were in the pipeline approved by the
Food and Drug Administration, and between 1977 and 1985 the stock went
up to about sixty-five a share, creating a significant increase in the resources
of the company and in shareholder value. (Unfortunately I only had about
200 shares, given to me as a token when I joined the Searle board.)

When Searle was sold to Monsanto in 1985, Dick Mahoney, Monsanto's

CEO, ran the meetings, which now alternated between Chicago and Saint Louis, the headquarters of Monsanto. The main thing Mahoney had in common with his predecessors was that they all enjoyed smoking very expensive cigars. Dick Mahoney, too, was an iron-fisted guy, but he wore his velvet glove well; he was a man of few words except when he thought something was important enough to enlarge on. The CEO for the Searle subsidiary, whom he recruited from Pfizer, became more of a leg-man than an autonomous CEO. The focus of board meetings during Rumsfeld's time tended to be financial and to a lesser extent programmatic (the board was made up of fellow CEOs of major corporations including Sears, the Harris Bank, and Esmark), whereas with Dick Mahoney the meetings were spent largely on programmatic and drug development affairs.

Rumsfeld had recruited Bob Shapiro as a legal counsel for G. D. Searle and Company, and after the company was sold to Monsanto, Mahoney made Shapiro head of the NutraSweet division, which he spun off from the immediate Searle subsidiary. Shapiro so impressed Mahoney that he recruited Shapiro to go to Monsanto headquarters in Saint Louis and be in charge of the agricultural division. What Mahoney was doing, in effect, was testing out Shapiro vis-à-vis some of his older colleagues at Monsanto to see which one would be a better successor. I am told that when Mahoney retired, he favored Bob Shapiro, which I think he probably has regretted since. Shapiro is a hard-nosed person, a very difficult guy to socialize with. I think some of the people at Monsanto have been concerned because he retained his residence in Chicago and commuted to Saint Louis. He was also not a good team leader: several of the operational people took early retirement and moved on. The Monsanto stock value dropped significantly from the time Mahoney was in charge. Shapiro favored putting all his eggs in the basket of genetically engineered agricultural products, and to create cash to do that, he sold the pharmaceutical component of Searle to Pharmacia Upjohn. Genetically engineered products are now a subject of worldwide controversy, and the market for them looks insecure and limited.

In 1991, at the age of sixty-five, I was retired from the board. In truth, I had become a little bored of the routine, and one of the lessons I learned was to recognize when I lost interest in a particular area of leadership and to make sure that I gave it up before my participation faltered. It was with that experience in mind that, in my fourth year as chairman of the board of Research!America, realizing that I would eventually tire of being responsible for the day-to-day running of the organization, I declined to be nominated for another term.

When Pearle Health Services was spun off from Searle in 1983, I was asked to serve on the Pearle board from 1983 to 1985. Their headquarters were in Dallas, so that meant a trek there every month or every other month for the board members, at which time we not only learned about Pearle Optical Services but were also outfitted with glasses for all occasions. They gave us eye examinations once or twice a year, and on one of those occasions it was discovered that I had glaucoma.

I came to love Dallas for a variety of reasons, including serving on that board, but also for my friendship with Caroline Hunt and her former husband, Buddy Schoellkopf, who provided the first round of helicopter service for Duke Life Flight. My work took me all over the nation, sometimes for activities directly related to the affairs of the Medical Center, sometimes for meetings and events that were only tangentially connected. Often there was no boundary between the personal and the public: I was able to nurture friendships and connections that directly benefited the Medical Center, and my national activities and the affairs of the Medical Center often led me into enduring friendships.

In 1966, when I was chair of the AAMC ways and means committee, I talked to both Tom Kinney and Dan Tosteson on my return from Washington about the committee's proposal to form three councils. They asked me if the AAMC was a serious venture, and I assured them that it was. Consequently, Tom Kinney became the first chair of the Council of Academic Societies, to be succeeded two years later by Dan Tosteson. In the meantime, in 1968, I became the first chairman of the new Council of Deans. So the three of us were in and out of Washington fairly regularly, and a special camaraderie developed.

The AAMC initiative led to other changes, particularly in Dan Tosteson's career from that point. Until that time, Tosteson had been very narrowly focused on the physiology of the membrane of the red blood cell. Suddenly, the whole world of medical education was at his feet. Shortly thereafter he began talking about the importance of changes in medical education and, not surprisingly, he began getting offers for deanships. I recall especially that he got an offer in the late seventies from the University of Pittsburgh, which he declined. About 1975–76, he received an offer to become dean of the medical school at the University of Chicago, which he accepted.

In the course of 1976 Derek Bok, the president of Harvard, was looking for a new medical dean to succeed the retiring Bob Ebert. Bok went out to Chicago and persuaded Dan Tosteson to return to his alma mater as dean of the Harvard Medical School. This really upset the people at Chicago,

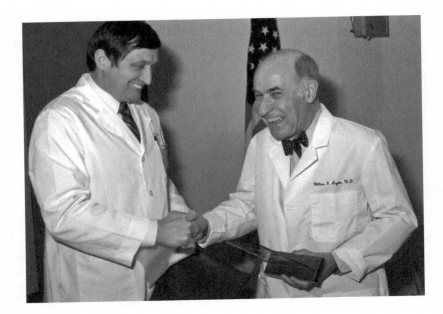

26   Dr. W. G. Anlyan visiting the University of Colorado School of Medicine with Dean Roy Schwarz, a long-time friend and subsequent vice president of the American Medical Association; currently president of the China Medical Board Foundation of New York. From personal archive of author.

and he was subsequently ostracized by both the Chicago faculty and the administrators, who were evidently extremely sensitive to having their ranks raided by Harvard.

In January 1977 I selected Dan to accompany me in a delegation to Egypt as guests of the ministers of health and education; our visit coincided with the food riots in Cairo, which resulted in our being cooped up in our hotel for two days. This gave me an occasion to have a beer with Dan and to ask him why he had made the transition to Harvard so soon after he had become dean and vice president at Chicago. He told me that he felt he had "conquered" the challenge at Chicago, especially of having a hospital and clinics under his authority. He really did not want to spend his time overseeing the clinics and hospital at the University of Chicago and that the challenge at Harvard, with the traditional basic sciences, seemed far greater. He did extremely well in his twenty years as the chief educational steward at the Harvard Medical School. Others in our delegation to Egypt included Dr. M. Roy Schwarz who was an associate dean in Seattle (currently president of the China Medical Board of New York, Inc.) and Dr. and Mrs. Kenneth Crispell (Ken was the vice president for health affairs at the University of Virginia).

One funny sidelight: After Dan arrived in Boston, he applied to the Country Club of Brookline and thought that with his title and position as dean of the Harvard Medical School he would be a shoo-in. They insisted on his getting some personal referrals, and so he had to call and ask me to write him a letter of support. He got in. Ironically, when he was at Duke he was fairly liberal socially and would never have entertained the thought of joining a club such as the Hope Valley Country Club, which was regarded as very conservative.

The delegation that I undertook with Dan Tosteson to Cairo points to another dimension of the work we did from our base at Duke. The Duke Medical Center was no longer a minor, unknown medical school and hospital in a small city in the southern United States. We had become influential players not only in the nation but also on the world stage.

13

THE CHANGING WORLD

CHANGES IN THE SCIENCE and practice of medicine, in information and communication, involved the world beyond the boundaries of the United States, in both developed and developing nations, and Duke was active on the international scene throughout the period of my tenure at the Medical Center and university. In addition to annual and semiannual trips abroad for informal meetings with colleagues in medical education or surgery, I was a member of several international delegations and played key roles in major meetings outside the United States.

In 1970, while I was a member of the Board of Regents of the National Library of Medicine, Marty Cummings, the director, asked if I would go on a consultation trip to Poland, Yugoslavia, and Israel. The purpose was to examine several projects the library was funding, primarily through the PL480 program, which essentially forgave the recipient country's debts by working off projects of mutual interest with the United States, in this case in the library communications field. I went with my wife, Connie, and the government was kind enough to accommodate us with first-class transportation all the way because of my bad back. (The staff person from the National Library also took his wife, but he booked her in tourist class, while he enjoyed the comforts of first-class travel all the way from the United States to Poland to Belgrade, Zagreb, and Tel Aviv. Not surprisingly, she divorced him shortly after they got back.)

In Poland we visited PL480 library programs not only in Warsaw but also in Krakow, where I also went to see the children's hospital, which I thought was outstanding. I had been warned before going to Poland not to tell any Polish jokes, but the moment I got there our hosts had a whole array of Polish jokes to tell us. I was very impressed by the spirit of the Polish people—their relatively spartan existence and poverty but good humor. Despite that relative poverty, they gave us full honors with multi-course meals and their finest wines. Equally impressive was our ambassador to Warsaw, who was fluent in Polish and highly respected by the Polish officials. We stayed at the main hotel downtown, the Europejski, but I had been warned that the rooms were bugged. Their eavesdropping system was not a very good one, and in the middle of the night it would hum, so we knew exactly where the microphones were.

In Yugoslavia we went to Belgrade and took a one-day trip to Zagreb. Then we flew to Tel Aviv, where our host was Dr. Moshe Prywes, then dean of the Hadassah Medical School. Dr. Prywes greeted us on arrival at the Tel Aviv airport. We spent most of the time in Jerusalem but also visited the medical school in Tel Aviv. I was particularly impressed with the synagogue in the Hadassah Medical School. They had donors' names on just about every nook and cranny of the facility. On a list of major donors I found the names of Mr. and Mrs. Eli Evans—he was the former mayor of Durham. When I got back a week after the trip, Eli was sitting next to me at a Duke football game, and I chided him for getting all his medical care at Duke but giving his money to Jerusalem. It was the Hadassah experience that convinced me of the importance of placing donor names on rooms, halls, and other facilities, as we continued to develop the Medical Center. We also visited Haifa and all the usual tourist stops, including the impressive Bahai Temple. We were privileged to have lunch with the Bahai "pope," who happened to be a convert from the midwestern United States. On leaving Israel I offered an invitation to Dr. Prywes to spend his upcoming sabbatical year at Duke, which he did.

On the way back from Jerusalem, we stopped in Rome for a few days, where we were the guests of Dr. Juan Castiglione, the chief of surgery at the Gemelli Hospital of the Vatican Medical School. In the course of the visit, Dr. and Mrs. Castiglione asked if we wanted to see the pope, and of course I did not say no, but I pointed out that whereas my wife, Connie, was a devout Catholic, I was a Protestant and that it might be an imposition, but they insisted that we should go on and see Pope Paul VI.

This was not our first audience with a pope or even with Paul VI. In 1959 Connie and I had gone to Castel Gandolfo to see Pope John XXIII. We were told to wear dark, solemn clothes, and the implication was that this would be a very personal visit. When we got there, we were part of a crowd

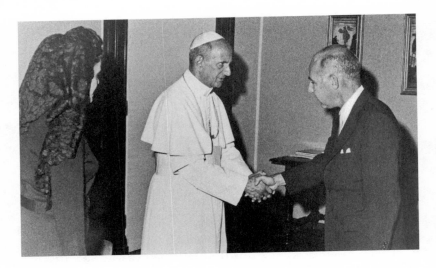

27 Dr. W. G. Anlyan and his wife, Connie, visiting Pope Paul VI at Castello Gondolfo, near Rome, 1970. Dr. Anlyan tried to convince Pope Paul that health workers throughout the world would provide a better matrix for World Peace than the ecumenical movement, composed as it was of religions that had been adversaries for centuries. From personal archive of author.

of twenty thousand people who were also visiting Pope John XXIII. As the pope was being carried in by the Swiss Guards, I suddenly felt a weight on my shoulders: a very small Italian nun had climbed up to get a better view, and from her perch she was yelling, "Il papa, il papa!" Obviously, getting a glimpse of the pope was the climax of her career.

My second visit with a pope was in 1963, when the International Cardiovascular Society met in Rome, and we were invited to a private audience with Pope Paul VI. Some of the devout Catholics among the surgeons ended up being invited to sit on the dais with the pope, whereas the other three thousand of us were in the hall on benches. One of the devout Catholics, Dr. Rollo Hanlon of Saint Louis, had not been permitted to sit on the dais because his tie was not conservative enough for the Swiss Guards, while his wife, a pediatrician who had borne twelve children, was given a seat.

During our 1970 trip the biggest black Fiat limousine I have ever seen drove up to the Hassler Hotel to pick us up and drive us to Castel Gandolfo. Once we got there, there was another crowd of twenty thousand.

But the guards came out, parted the crowds and let our limousine through the inner gates, where we were greeted by a butler in formal regalia who took us up to a second-floor antechamber. Shortly behind us, another big black limousine had driven up and deposited a monsignor; he too came into the antechamber, announcing that he was Father Koveny from Cork, Ireland, and was the number 2 English-speaking priest at the Vatican. He apologized that the number 1 English-speaking priest was on vacation, so he was substituting. I asked him why he was there, and he said he was to be the interpreter between Pope Paul VI's Italian and my English. When he found out that I spoke French fluently, he said, "The pope also speaks French so I'll stand in the background. If either one of you stumbles in the conversation, I'll chime in."

Fifteen minutes later, Connie and I sat across a small desk from Pope Paul VI and carried on a wonderful conversation about the fact that health workers, and particularly doctors, would be a better avenue for world peace than theologians, priests, and ministers. My visit to Israel had reminded me of all the conflicts caused by religious differences in the past two thousand years. At one point I thought that the pope agreed with me, because this was at the height of the ecumenical movement for world peace. I invited him to come to the AAMC meeting in Washington later that fall. He thanked me and said that since his travel was limited, he would send an encyclical. I thought the subject would be world peace and what physicians and health workers could do to enhance the ecumenical movement. Instead, a week before the AAMC meeting, where I was chairman of the assembly that year, he sent an encyclical decrying the evils of birth control and abortion. We did not announce the fact that we had an encyclical because we did not want to embarrass anyone.

The meeting with Pope Paul VI lasted about twenty-five minutes and was very cordial, and as we parted we shook hands. As we were about halfway down a long hallway on our way out, a short Italian photographer who had taken pictures of our meeting chased me down and asked me how many copies of the pictures I wanted. At that point I did not know if I should ask for one or a hundred, so I just said, "The usual." Next day, there was a package at the hotel from the official Vatican photographer with five prints of the picture, along with a rather substantial bill for services rendered.

In 1972, as part of the more formal national interest in other countries, I started the first bilateral conference between medical education counterparts in Britain and the United States; the conference was supported by the United Kingdom's Nuffield Foundation and the Commonwealth Foundation of New York. People such as Dr. John A. D. Cooper, president of the AAMC, and Alex McMahon, president of the American Hospital Association, were among those from the United States; on the British side, perhaps the most notable participant was Dr. John Lister, who for twenty-eight years wrote the monthly column "By the London Post" in the *New England Journal of Medicine*.

Meetings subsequently became trilateral with the inclusion of Canada and continue to take place every couple of years, rotating among the three countries. The American leader has become Dr. Roger Bulger, who had been at Duke in allied health education. Previous to that he was an associate dean at the University of Washington in Seattle; for many years now he has been the full-time president of the Association of Academic Health Centers (AAHC). The heads in England and Canada are the new leaders of their medical education associations. The last two trilateral conferences I attended were in Irvine, California (1991) and Oxford, England (1994).

In April 1975 I took up a position as a visiting professor at the American University of Beirut, which entailed giving multiple lectures, including a presentation on United States medical education at the twenty-fifth Middle East Medical Assembly. I followed the prime minister of Lebanon, who was accompanied to the podium by a platoon of armed soldiers. In my opening remarks I apologized for not bringing my own escort—little did I know that exactly two weeks later Beirut would blow up with the beginning of the civil war. My host was Dr. Sam Asper, the dean at the American University. I had known him for a long time in his position as a professor of surgical pathology at Johns Hopkins—particularly when I was recruiting Dave Sabiston in 1964.

The American University of Beirut is a fine institution. Its medical alumni returning for the April 1975 meeting held key positions in universities from Turkey to Ethiopia and extended in the Orient to Singapore. I was so impressed that I had the passing thought of suggesting to my children that it was the place to spend a semester abroad. The city of Beirut and the Saint George's Hotel where I stayed were charming and obviously at the crossroads of the world. The many wonderful meals of Lebanese food reminded me of the Alexandria of my youth.

En route to Beirut, I had attended a Macy Foundation conference in Mas D'Artigny (just north of Nice, France) for several days. I found out that there was a direct Air France flight from Nice to Cairo. Since the Macy conference finished on Friday morning and I wasn't due in Beirut till Monday afternoon, I arranged to fly to Cairo to visit my only living relative in Egypt—Uncle Leon, who still lived in Alexandria. Leon met me at the Cairo airport. I spent Friday night at the Sheraton Hotel in the center of a city where the cars honking extended to the early morning hours. The next day I looked forward with great anticipation to seeing Alexandria again for the first time in over thirty years since my departure in August 1943. What a shock I had driving into town to see all the once-beautiful houses and streets, including the one we had lived in, so dilapidated. Apparently when Nasser ousted Farouk, he instituted rent controls, so that there was no incentive for landlords to maintain the quality of buildings—apartments and houses that once matched some of the elegant quarters of Paris.

I checked into the Cecil Hotel in downtown Alexandria. There was no other hotel of any substance in 1975; the Palestine Hotel in Montaza, where I have stayed in subsequent visits, was not built till later. The clerk at the check-in desk at the Cecil greeted me with the gusto of an old friend. He told me how fortunate I was, because he was assigning me General Bernard Montgomery's suite, which the general had occupied during the North African Campaign of World War II. The suite turned out to be a shabby and noisy one directly on the Corniche (the road that runs along the Alexandria waterfront and Eastern Harbor). Cockroaches appeared after dark. About 6:00 P.M. I went down to the lobby to wait for Leon to pick me up for dinner. While sitting across from the registration desk, I watched a gentleman checking in. The same desk clerk greeted him and confided that luckily he was going to be in General Montgomery's old suite.

My uncle was very gracious. He and his wife gave me a royal reception for the next forty-eight hours, visiting his private clubs and the best that Alexandria could offer under the circumstances. He got me to my Cairo-Beirut flight in time on Monday morning.

The only other occasion when I occupied the quarters of a former commanding general, they were the real thing. It was in Paris in the early 1990s. I was a guest of Henry Carnegie, the legal counsel of the Aga Khan, who owned the Meurice Hotel. They graciously put us up in the elegant suite that had been occupied by the commanding German general during the Occupation of Paris. One morning, while calling my Duke office sitting at the beautiful desk in the living room, I noted that there was a plaque commemorating the fact that this was the desk on which the general had signed the German surrender of Paris in 1944. He was also the general who refused Hitler's orders to blow up all those beautiful bridges on the Seine River before the surrender.

Starting in 1975 I made four visits to Japan as a guest of the Japanese gov-

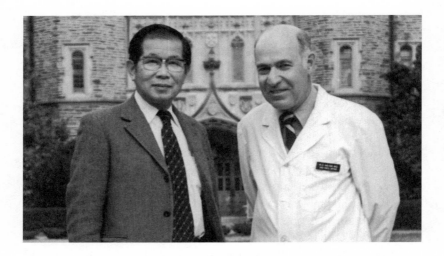

28   Dr. Shigeaki Hinohara, chairman of the board, Saint Luke's International Hospital, Tokyo, Japan, on one of his frequent visits to Duke University. Dr. Hinohara has been a pioneer in health maintenance in Japan for several decades. His father graduated from Trinity College in 1904, and his son Tommy was a postdoctoral fellow in cardiology at Duke. DUMC Photography.

ernment. On my first trip, I was a guest lecturer at the Life Planning Center in Tokyo, and my host was Dr. Shigeaki Hinohara, the head of the center. The center is something like an HMO, giving comprehensive wellness advice and care. Dr. Hinohara was supported in this endeavor by Mr. Sasakawa, a war criminal who had been spared by General MacArthur so that he could help reorganize Japanese industry after World War II. Mr. Sasakawa was a multimillionaire, partly as a result of organizing the betting on motorboat races in Tokyo Bay. He had put some of his money in a foundation that supported the Life Planning Center. They had an annual symposium, with guests from the United States, Canada, and Great Britain.

Dr. Hinohara's father had been a student at Trinity College, the precursor of Duke University, in 1904. He had been sent here by Methodist missionaries, and because he was so poor, he was referred to as a "Japanese waif" in archival materials that I have consulted. He roomed in the house of Dr. Flowers, then dean of Trinity College (and later president of Duke University), because he could not afford the room rent in Trinity. Dr. Hinohara had never forgotten the fact that his father was an alumnus of Duke University, and we have had a long-standing, very cordial relationship with him. He has lectured at Duke, and at one point, he asked me if his son Tommy, after graduating from the University of Tokyo Medical School, could come to Duke to be trained in medicine. As a preliminary to his coming here, and with Jim Wyngaarden's help, we had Tommy Hinohara spend a year in Okinawa learning English, and then another year in Montreal. Subsequently, he came to Duke as a fellow in cardiology. Tommy married a Japanese woman, but they decided they did not want to go back and live in the feudal society of Japan. They are now located in Palo Alto, where he is in a group practicing cardiology, doing extremely well. So we have a long-standing relationship with the family, which recently signed an agreement to fund a scholarship at Duke University Medical School in the name of the three generations of Hinoharas at Duke.

The trip to Tokyo in 1975 was very interesting, because we landed at Hanada, the old airport, since Narita, the international airport, was still under construction. Greeting me at the airport were Dr. Hinohara, as well as the deans of the five medical schools in the Tokyo area. Each one of the deans gave me a gift, including magnificent, 150-year-old artist's sketches of the road between Kyoto and Tokyo. The hosts put me up at the Crown Prince Hotel and gave me two large manila envelopes filled with my honorarium, since at that time Japanese bills were very large and got bigger the higher the denomination. I had to rent two deposit boxes to store the money, since it included my airfare. After two and a half days I had to dash back to New York, because the bond issue for constructing the new North Division of Duke hospital was going to be rated, and I had to be present when Moody's and Standard & Poor interviewed the staff to determine our rating. (Moody's gave our bonds an A1 rating, Standard & Poor's an AA.)

The Japanese medical schools are divided into two clusters: private schools and public schools. The best schools are the public ones, especially the University of Tokyo. The private schools were created to serve rich youngsters, particularly the sons and daughters of physicians who could not compete to get into the public system. Tuition is extremely high in the private schools, but this is obviously recouped in the first few years of practice. Most of the research is done in the public system. The hospitals are immaculate, and, at least from the point of surgery, the surgeons are every bit as good as their American counterparts.

That first trip to Japan was a brief one, but I have been back on other occasions to lecture, and the Japanese were always delightful. On one of the trips, we were taken for a weekend to a very lovely old Japanese hotel at the foot of Mount Fuji; on another trip we were taken to Kyoto, which I

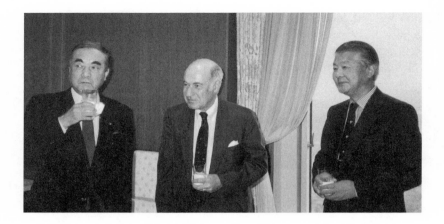

29   Dr. W. G. Anlyan with Prime Minister Nakasone and Duke alumnus Hideo Ishihara, head of the Goldman Sachs branch in Tokyo, 1978. From personal archive of author.

found charming. I had a hard time ignoring my guilt feelings over the fact that Japan was the only country whose people had experienced an atom bomb explosion. The Japanese I met were very stoic about it, and the subject never came up in social conversation. I also had a hard time sitting on cushions for fourteen-course meals. I would stack a number of pillows to sit up as high as possible, to ease the pain in my back and hips. The first time I experienced such a marathon meal, I had no way of guessing after the third or fourth course how many more were coming. And I never did develop a taste for sake.

In October 1975 I had the privilege of being head of the Duke delegation to visit the People's Republic of China for three weeks. In July 1972 President Terry Sanford called me while I was hosting the Duke Medical Symposium in Atlantic Beach, North Carolina. It was 7:30 A.M. when the telephone rang. "Do you want to go with a Duke delegation to China?" he asked. My response was "Do you mean Taiwan?" because the United States did not have diplomatic relations with Maoist China. He reassured me that it was the real China. Since I had the utmost trust in Terry Sanford's abilities, I agreed to go "when and if" the trip occurred. In May 1975 Terry heard from an intermediary in Ottawa that we would be invited for three weeks starting in mid-October of 1975.

As October approached, the twelve-person delegation was identified. In addition to Terry and Mrs. Sanford, it included Duke trustee Jack White-head and his wife, Betsy; Ken and Judy Pye (Ken was dean of the law school, after a stint as chancellor); and members of the faculty, staff, and students. However, closer to departure time, Terry had become interested in running for the presidency of the United States. Reluctantly he decided to forego China; Margaret Rose Sanford would go as the "First Lady" of the delegation, and as the next ranking senior university officer, I would head up the delegation.

The only suggestion I made to the delegation was as follows: "If you wish, please let me know of any special medical problems you may have. Since I've never been to China and don't know the quality of medical care, let us avoid any surprises. Please bring your own regular medications as well as your favorite booze." Unbeknownst to one member of the delegation who had benign prostatic hypertrophy, I did pack a few urethral catheters that were never needed. There were no other medical problems.

Our rendezvous was the Peninsula Hotel in Hong Kong, the only point of entry to the People's Republic. At the suggestion of Ken Pye, Jack Whitehead and I had brought along our tennis racquets and tennis balls in anticipation of two days of leisure in Hong Kong. Unfortunately it rained, and the equipment remained unused. At the designated time we boarded the train in front of the Peninsula Hotel for the two-hour ride to Canton. We were met at the Canton train station by the number 2 head of the Chinese In-tourist delegation and his staff. For the next three weeks, we were completely in their charge.

On each occasion, there were six or seven cars for our delegation and their staff. It was made clear that Mrs. Sanford and I would be in the number 1 car with the number 2 In-tourist gentleman. The number 1 car varied from location to location. At the larger communities, it was a Chinese replica of the Russian Ziv. The rest of the delegation followed us in lesser vehicles. During bouts of rain, it became apparent that the defrosting system of their latest limos could not cope with the humidity. The driver would hand each one of us a rag to wipe our windows so we could see the surrounding countryside.

In Canton (now Guangzhou) we witnessed two eye operations performed under acupuncture. To my pleasant surprise, all the delegation attended and nobody fainted. In both cases, the patient walked into the operating room. He got on the operating table. The anesthesiologist appeared. She "prepped" the area surrounding the appropriate eye with antiseptic. She then picked up the jar containing the silver acupuncture needles and with her bare fingers selected two needles. She introduced one needle into the infraorbital nerve just below the eye and the second in the supraorbital nerve groove above the eye socket. She connected the two needles to a machine via electric wires. At this point the eye surgeon came in; he was appropriately gowned and gloved. Within about fifteen minutes the minor ophthalmic operation was completed. At the conclusion, the patient would sit up and shake the surgeon's hand before walking out to his room. In view of the lack of sterile technique, my question to the anesthesiologist was "What is your incidence of infections?" She said they never had any! I later found that that there was no follow-up.

From Canton we flew to Shanghai. Thereafter, we visited Soochow, Nanking, with our final stop in Beijing. That last leg was accomplished by an overnight train from Nanking to Beijing. The accommodations on the train were Victorian. The toilets were acceptable for the men but the women in the delegation had trouble coping with the lack of appropriate facilities. Three of the ladies shared a compartment, and Jack Whitehead, Ken Pye, and I shared another. We flipped for the bunks. I got the single bunk on one side. Jack had the high bunk on the other side. One of the two, either Jack or Ken snored loudly all night. So much for old-fashioned sleeper accommodations on trains.

In Nanking I developed a classic case of the flu. While the rest of the delegation went on a two-day side trip, I remained alone in my hotel room. Three times a day a young man would show up with a meal. By the third day, the food smelled somewhat rancid. For a humidifier, I would turn on the hot shower in the tub to steam up the room. In any event I survived; members of the delegation loaned me their favorite novels, which I read during those long hours.

Beijing was thrilling. We were greeted there by Dr. George Hatem, Chairman Mao's personal physician. A native of Roanoke Rapids, North Carolina, he was a first-generation Lebanese-American. He had gone to Switzerland to medical school and on completing his studies in the 1930s, had decided to return to the United States via the Orient. Instead of returning home he stayed in China and linked up with the Maoist regime. He became a devout follower of Chairman Mao and married a Chinese woman who produced educational movies. Hatem did not return to the United States and North Carolina until just before his death, on October 3, 1988.

The year 1975 was the nadir of the Maoist revolution. Yet George and everyone else in positions of authority echoed the party line, "Everything is fine!" Candidates for medical school were being selected by the rulers of the commune. Instead of four years of college, followed by four of medical school and three to five years of internship and residency training, as we do it in the United States, the Chinese students went through a total of three years. The older pre-Maoist physicians were disgusted but reluctant to voice their opinions. And then there were "barefoot doctors," who in three months were trained to screen people within an assigned geographic area for potential medical care. They also advised on preventive and contraceptive care.

On one Sunday afternoon in Beijing, Jack Whitehead and I agreed to tour a "traditional hospital." There were 231 in-patients, and Jack and I visited each one. Those patients receiving "traditional care," consisting mainly of herbal medicine, were divided into two groups in our judgment. Those in group 1 were experiencing "placebo" care. For example, a twenty-six-year-old married man with two children was being treated for peptic ulcers of the stomach and duodenum. On his herbal medication he was vastly improved over a two-week period—confirming the old British saying that ulcers are caused by the family or the job. If sequestered, they will get better. Needless to say, there were no controls.

Group 2 looked much more promising. We saw, for example, three young women, diagnosed as having "leukemia." On herbal therapy for three months, their white blood cell counts had (it was claimed) come down to normal levels. We only had access to numerical data, and neither of us would have been competent to review hematologic blood smears. All three patients looked well. As a follow-up, on my return to the United States, I urged some pharmacological groups to go to China and investigate what might be the active ingredient. In the back of my mind, I had the example of heart medicines derived from foxglove (digitalis) and the synthetic analogs created thereafter.

Returning from Beijing to the United States was a challenge. On one of my few calls to my office from Beijing, it became apparent that I needed to be in Durham at least two days earlier than planned for an important meeting regarding the new hospital. I asked my In-tourist companion if it might be possible for me to change my itinerary and fly directly from Beijing to Tokyo and on to the United States. On that particular day there was an Iran Air flight scheduled that flew to Tokyo. This would obviate my going with the rest of the delegation back to Canton and taking with them the train to Hong Kong and then the long, scheduled flight back to the United States. I had cleared the request with the rest of our delegation. My In-tourist companion got approval for the change.

Early on that Sunday morning I was driven to the Beijing airport. The young Chinese man at the official airline counter was surrounded by a group of teenagers who were learning how the job was done. Much to my surprise, the agent refused to check my luggage beyond Tokyo to San Francisco on the connecting Pan Am flight at Tokyo's Hanada airport. The connection was thirty-five minutes. I tried to explain to the agent that time would not permit my disembarking at Tokyo, going through customs, retrieving my luggage, and rechecking it. He refused. "Why?" I asked— Because Pan Am was an American airline and China did not have formal diplomatic relations with the United States. Throughout this argument, my In-tourist guide stood by speechless because the agent was exerting his authority in the presence of the group of students.

With a sigh of desperation, I boarded the Iran Air plane knowing full well that Iran Air was closely linked in its operations with Pan Am. As the plane took off, I called for the chief steward. I explained the situation to him and added that I was an old friend of Dr. Farouk Saidi, the shah's surgeon, who had trained in part at Duke. If the steward could help me, I would write a letter of commendation to Dr. Saidi. The steward said when we left Chinese airspace he would radio ahead to Tokyo for instructions.

When the Iran Air captain announced that we had left China's airspace, I experienced a spontaneous sigh of relief. Fortunately our arrival in Tokyo was on time. The steward made sure that I would be the first to disembark. As the cabin door opened a Japanese gentleman in a blue blazer came in, grabbed me by the arm and led me down the steps to a limousine. He introduced himself as the general manager of Pan Am at Hanada airport. Shortly thereafter my baggage appeared and was put in the car. We cut across Hanada airport to the waiting Pan Am 747. I made it with five minutes to spare.

As I reflect on the three-week visit to China, I recall two other interesting experiences. For the first few days, at every institution we visited (and we saw as many as four or five a day), the first twenty minutes was always consumed by a monologue in Chinese on the glories of the Maoist Revolution. This was repeated in English, phrase by phrase by the interpreter. It became a major source of dismay and dissatisfaction with all members of our delegation. We agreed to do something about it. Our solution was fairly simple. We knew that many of the hotel rooms were bugged, especially mine as head of the delegation. Each evening we had about forty-five minutes when we would be left alone before being escorted to dinner. We called those breaks "the Ping Hour"—"ping" meant ice in Chinese. We ordered ice for drinks; each person who still had a bottle of spirits would bring it to share with the delegation. In Shanghai, I was given a nice suite in the French hotel where President Nixon and his entourage had stayed. The members of our delegation became very vocal about how ridiculous the preludes were. That afternoon we had visited the Shanghai Municipal Hospital and had met with Dr. Chen, the renowned orthopedic surgeon who had reattached the first severed arm in China. Even though Dr. Chen was fluent in English he had to give his Maoist recitation in Chinese. During the rest of our visit with Dr. Chen, he and I conversed privately in English. Much to our delight the preludes ceased the next morning.

The other interesting experience was our final Sunday afternoon in Beijing, which was spent with the minister of education. In my comments, I remarked that we had not seen any programs that produced "cookie cutters" —meaning teachers who would educate and prepare the next generation. We had been warned before we left the United States that when our Chinese hosts got uncomfortable with our queries, they would wander off into Maoist philosophy. Our minister of education was no exception—so I backed off.

Six weeks later in December of 1975 there was an article in the *New York Times* with a Hong Kong byline stating that the minister of education had been removed for advocating the "production of cookie cutters." Three months later, the *New York Times* reported that he had died. Should I have felt guilty?

Many years later, in September 2002, my wife, Alex, and I were invited to visit five medical centers in China under the sponsorship of the China Medical Board Foundation and its president, Mr. Roy Schwarz. (The China Medical Board Foundation is a nonprofit organization started in 1913 as an offshoot of the Rockefeller Foundation to assist medical education in China; in recent years it has given China approximately $10 milion a year in grants, which translates to a purchasing power of $200 million a year in the United States.) The state of Chinese medical education and health care in 2002 could not have been more different. In the course of the trip, we visited Beijing, Chunking, Shanghai, and Sian, and saw how extensively the medical system has been modernized.

The Chinese aspire to make the level of care equal to that available in the United States and are proud that biomedical scientists who had emigrated to the United States are returning to China. Biomedical engineering is already very advanced. In the leading medical schools in China, medical education now entails seven to eight years before residency training.

The only remnant of training in traditional Chinese medicine is a block of forty to fifty hours during the preresidency period; traditional medicine is taught for historical reasons and (as one medical professor put it) for foreign tourists. At least in the cities we visited, science, medicine, engineering, computer and communication systems, architecture, and transportation are now much more comparable with what we have in the United States. China has come a long way since my first visit there in 1975.

In March 1976 I traveled again to Poland, a more formal visit this time, under the auspices of the United States Bureau of Health Manpower. I was part of a larger group, including Ken Endicott, Roy Schwarz, and John Cooper, who was then president of the AAMC. We spent most of the time in Warsaw, looking at their programs of medical education, and then went to Krakow. The trip back to Warsaw was a twelve-hour bus ride through a March snow blizzard. I recalled with nostalgia my trip in 1970, which was a one-hour plane ride between Krakow and Warsaw.

On this visit, we were housed in the official residence for visiting dignitaries in Warsaw, and once again the rooms were bugged. There had been notable progress in the six years since 1970 in the construction of new hotels and cleaning things up; the Polish people were on the road to recovery. One of the most shocking sites we visited was the old town of Warsaw. The Germans bombed and burned this area over a period of six months, while the Russians stood by across the Vistula River and let the destruction go on. On the plus side, this has given the Polish government the opportunity to rebuild old Warsaw, and there were interesting innovations such as using a single hot-water system, which also provided heat for the buildings of the old town.

Late in 1976 Ken Endicott, the chief of the Bureau of Health Manpower in the Department of Health, Education and Welfare, asked me to head up a delegation to Cairo, which we scheduled for January 1977. I had known Ken for many years when he was at the NIH. In 1972 Endicott, Russ Nelson, president of Johns Hopkins Hospital, and I had been on a tour of England and France on our way to a Macy Conference in The Hague. The trip to the Netherlands was complicated by a one-day pilots' strike, forcing us to rent a car to drive from Paris to The Hague. The concierge at the Hotel Lancaster in Paris misdirected us on the way out of Paris, so we kept going in circles on the road known as the "peripherique," which circled Paris. After going by the Eiffel Tower twice, we admitted we were lost. We finally pulled into a fire station, where the chief, identifiable by his immense abdomen, was very sympathetic and assigned one of the younger firemen to escort us out of Paris in great style with what must have been a 1920s fire wagon. On the trip, our car was driven alternately by Nelson and Endicott, both of whom turned out to be old farmer families from North Dakota, so the conversation in the car as we drove through the vast countryside was a discussion by the two farm boys of the crops they saw.

We arrived in Egypt during the second week of January 1977. We were the guests of the minister of health and the minister of education, to try to help them improve medical education. I was allowed to select my own delegation, so I picked Dr. Kenneth Crispell, vice president of the University of Virginia, who chose to take his wife, Marge, along with us; Dr. Roy Schwarz, at that time associate dean at the University of Washington at Seattle; and Dr. Dan Tosteson, who was in limbo between the University of Chicago School of Medicine and Harvard Medical School. Our group was accompanied by a U.S. Air Force lieutenant colonel, serving as security officer, and we were housed at the Nile Hilton Hotel. In the middle of our official visit, on a Tuesday evening, we were the dinner guests of the two ministers in one of King Farouk's former palaces. The dinner was interrupted several times by phone calls from Sadat to his two ministers, who had to excuse themselves periodically to take the calls. After dinner, the minister of health gave Dan Tosteson and me a ride back to the Nile Hilton and somebody threw a rock through one of the car windows, which fortunately missed all three of us. This was the beginning of the food riots in Egypt.

We were asked to remain quarantined in the hotel, a request we obeyed, especially after the original driver assigned to us went outdoors to check on the curfew and was shot through the thigh by the police. So we stayed in the hotel until things quieted down. Our Air Force escort suggested that we each pack a small bag in the event we needed to evacuate; he would lead us the few blocks to the American embassy, if that were to become necessary. The Crispells were scared to death and wanted the embassy to ship them out immediately, but we persuaded them to stay on. Two days later, the riots had been quelled, and we were taken to the Cairo airport and shipped to Luxor for the weekend. By the time we got back from there, normal life had resumed in Cairo, and we completed our mission.

Before we had left the States, Ken Endicott had indicated to me what I could promise the two ministers in terms of help from the United States. High on my list was a health sciences library in Cairo that could network to all of the schools in Egypt and perhaps also hook up with the health sciences library in Jerusalem, so that it would serve as another form of dialogue between Egypt and Israel. (This was before Sadat and Begin signed the peace accord in the Rose Garden.) And so, at a full press conference, with the two ministers present, I made the promises that Ken Endicott had told me I could make.

On the way home, we stopped in Rome for two nights to unwind. There, we learned that the new government, with Joe Califano as the new secretary of health, education, and welfare, had fired Endicott. When we finally made it back to the United States, we did not know to whom we should report. It took about ten months, with some help from Dr. Juanita Kreps, the Duke economist who was secretary of commerce by this time, to find out to whom I should present an official account of the promises made to the Egyptian government.

In the meantime, I was getting letters from the two ministers asking what had happened. The confusion of changing administrations and not having a minister of health nor, at that time, of education, in our own government was a real handicap. I worked on the library project until 1992, when I took my next-to-last trip to Cairo. I ran into two buzz saws. On the American side, I discovered that the U.S. Agency for International Development (USAID) was very, very protective of its own interests and did not want to take on any new projects, particularly if the ideas belonged to somebody else. With the help of Dr. Donald Lindberg, the new director of the National Library of Medicine, we could have overcome that problem; as a matter of fact, Don sent one or two emissaries to Cairo to help with the spadework. At the Cairo end, the problem was with the minister of health and the dean of the Cairo University School of Medicine, as to who would be responsible for the base operation of the network.

In March 1978, through intermediaries who knew Duke University Hospital and me, we were invited to go to Tehran to advise the shah on the management structure of the Imperial Medical Center of Iran, which was just being constructed. Beforehand, around Christmas 1977, I had sent John Shytle, our assistant vice president for business and finance, with Ike Robinson, director of the hospital, and Ruby Wilson, dean of the Nursing School, to Tehran to assess whether we should have a relationship and if it was worth my while to go over. The group recommended that I visit in March 1978. All their travel was paid by the Iranian government.

Accordingly I went, traveling via Switzerland. At the invitation of Betty Dumaine of Pinehurst, I first visited the Princess Mother of Thailand in Gstaad, where she spent each winter (I was on the board of her charitable foundation). The subsequent Swissair flight from Geneva to Tehran was listed as having one stop—they did not tell you where that stop would be. It turned out to be Baghdad. We left off four or five passengers at the Baghdad airport and immediately took off again, without taking on any others. We landed in Tehran at 1:30 A.M., to be met by the shah's personal physician, Dr. Chuck Samy. He had been a classmate of Bob Whalen's, the Duke cardiologist, at Cornell Medical College. Whalen told me that Samy had been top of his class, by a large margin. Dr. Samy took us to the Intercontinental Hotel, and from the airport to the hotel we went through every red light in town. I thought that maybe after midnight they permitted that in Tehran, but the next day he did the same thing at nine in the morning. The Iranians were probably some of the worst drivers I have ever seen. At the Intercontinental we were put on the top floor, half of which was dedicated to a complete residence—not just a suite—for visiting prime ministers and the like. Tehran was almost a crossroads of the world for university and medical educators who were seeking money from the shah. One evening we were taken to a sumptuous feast at one of the private clubs and met a lot of familiar people, including many representatives of the Ivy League schools.

We spent about three hours with the shah of Iran. On that occasion, Fred and Barbara Cleaveland were with us; he was then provost of Duke University. Fred and I, with the permission of Terry Sanford, presented the shah with an academic robe as a token of our esteem, and we gave him a certificate making him an honorary alumnus of Duke. An old Iranian surgeon friend had suggested that Duke grant the shah an honorary degree, but we did not think it would be a good move, since this would have had to go through all the academic hoops at Duke, and the shah even at that time was a controversial figure (nor had we forgotten the brouhaha when Dr. Davison had wanted to give an honorary degree to then vice president Nixon).

After looking over the plans for the Imperial Medical Center in Tehran, we agreed to assist the shah with the establishment of the administrative structure. We would also accept students in our Program in Health Administration as part of the deal. Because I was busily writing out a contract, which I had never done before, nor have since, I decided to skip a one-day side trip to Ishfahan, an old and very interesting place. I thought I could always see that later, since it seemed that I would be going back to Iran at least every six months or so to supervise the project. Of course, I have never been able to get to Ishfahan, even though I still have the ticket for the trip.

It was a tremendous surprise to me when, eight months later, the shah was deposed. At the time of my visit, I thought he was very secure in his position. Immediately after the overthrow, Dr. Samy packed his family onto a plane and took off from Iran, leaving behind numerous beautiful and extremely well-furnished houses. He appeared in my office in 1979, looking for a job as an internist. I believe he ended up at Cornell, although Jim Wyngaarden, who was then our chairman of medicine, looked seriously at the possibility of offering him a position. In the course of that visit, I asked Dr. Samy if the communists had been responsible for the downfall of the shah; he said no, not at all, that it was the policies of President Carter, who had leaned on the shah for more and more human rights concessions, as a result of which a sufficient number of political prisoners had been released to form a critical mass that could overthrow the shah. We had some money on deposit from Iran and this got negotiated to finalize the payments for at least one of the students in our health administration program.

In 1980 I was invited to visit Saudi Arabia. The invitation came from Roy Schwarz, at that time dean of the University of Colorado Medical School. He put together a small group including John Cooper, president of the AAMC, and Robert Van Citters, the dean at the University of Washington. When I got to Riyadh I noted that they knew everything about the North Division of our hospital because Hellmuth, Obata & Kassebaum (HOK), the architectural firm that designed our facility, had competed for the job of designing the new campus of the University of Riyadh as well as the international airport that was to be built in that city. The cover of the brochure HOK had prepared to pitch for the contract featured the front of our Duke Hospital North Division.

When we arrived, the international airport was still in Dahran, and one took a commuter flight to Riyadh. It became apparent to us that the Saudis do not adhere to posted schedules for their flights: they seem to leave whenever it is convenient (for them), so you had to keep an eye on when the flight was going to leave. In spite of the fact that we had official United States passports, customs went through our luggage very thoroughly, looking for liquor or pornography. For ten days we abstained from any alcoholic beverages. The U.S. Embassy, located in Jeddah, was kind enough to arrange for our ambassador to spend a day with us, and he laughed at our stories. It was particularly ironic because one day we visited the King Faisal Hospital, the royal hospital in a compound and grounds of its own, used exclusively by members of the royal family. We discovered the most common single cause for hospitalization was alcoholism. Furthermore, they falsified the records so there was no record of the experience. I found this pretty hard to take.

At dinner we would be served nonalcoholic wine, which tasted awful, at a price of about eighty dollars a bottle.

The Saudis were also very tough on women, particularly American women, who could do nothing but stay in their hotel rooms; they could not go swimming in the outdoor pool or play tennis, and they could only go out accompanied by their husbands, despite the fact that they were in chauffeur-driven cars. Some of them were pinched in the marketplace, because the perception of American women was that they were promiscuous, an impression the Saudis got from the movies. I would say that if there is one country I would not be enthusiastic about revisiting it would be Saudi Arabia, and I certainly would never take any American woman—including my wife—to that country. Subsequent to that ten-day visit, we developed some relationships that accelerated considerably during the time of Dr. Ralph Snyderman, my successor as head of the Medical Center, when the mother of one of the leading princes came to Duke for surgery.

On the return trip, John Cooper and I once again took the commuter flight from Riyadh to Dahran and then boarded a Pan Am 747 nonstop flight to New York. With us on the plane were four Saudi Arabian princesses, dressed in black robes, their faces covered. About two minutes after the no-smoking sign was turned off, the young princesses disappeared into the toilets and came back in sports shirts and jeans, and proceeded to smoke and drink champagne for the fourteen hours to New York.

On other trips, taking the Concorde in Paris on my way back from World Health Organization meetings in Geneva, it was not unusual to see a Saudi prince in the lounge before the flight, surrounded by bodyguards who were drinking orange or tomato juice, while the prince downed one Scotch after another.

I succeeded John Cooper on the committee on parasitic diseases of the WHO, serving from 1980 to 1984. The WHO is composed of a variety of regions as well as countries in the world. I was one of thirty-five people on this committee, and in my position I represented North America, both the United States and Canada. Parasitic diseases represent the biggest health problem in the world, particularly in the developing countries, and therefore the organization devotes a considerable amount of time to that issue. The twice-yearly meetings would usually last three or four days.

Although I had permission to fly on the Concorde to Paris, I would take a nonstop Swissair flight from New York to Geneva, get there at 7 A.M., booking my hotel room from the previous night so I could take a shower and shave, and get to the meeting by 9 A.M. I functioned reasonably well during the morning, but after lunch I would find it extremely hard to stay awake in the meeting. Falling asleep could have been embarrassing, because all the countries around the table were very interested in the reaction of the North American delegate in the various deliberations: it was not a good thing to doze off while they were talking. Most of the business was conducted in either English or French, so I did not have to resort to earphones and translations. I was selected for the position not because I knew much about parasitic diseases, but because I knew the medical education and research system in the United States and Canada. The same holds true of my predecessor, John Cooper, who was a biochemist, but who also clearly knew the channels for any issue that came up where the United States could be helpful.

One of the problems I encountered at the WHO was that the United States had not paid its dues for a considerable time. At least once a year the director general would invite me to have a cup of coffee with him in his office on the top floor of the WHO building. He would ask me to prod the U.S. government, which of course I was in no position to do. All I could— and did—do was transmit the message through official channels.

The experience in Geneva was very rewarding since it gave me the time on weekends to tour the surrounding countryside, and occasionally I would rent a car and go to Lausanne for a Sunday meal or to visit Chamonix and the Mont Blanc area. I found Switzerland to be very livable. Life was expensive, but as long as you stuck to nonluxury items and used the streetcars and buses, it was not too bad. Taxis were very expensive, as were wine, liquor, and good food. I would stay at Geneva's Hotel President. A sheik from one of the Arab states was generally in residence when I was there; I never did find out which one of the emirates he was from, but his bodyguards were slumped in armchairs in the hallway on the same floor I was on. Whenever he had dinner in the hotel dining room, his bodyguards were at two other separate tables with a clear view of him. I used to ask the hotel manager when I left whether he wanted to be paid in riyals or Swiss francs. I almost get nostalgic now when I fly over Geneva and think of the days I spent there.

Among my favorite places in Europe are the cities of Oxford and Cambridge. I have had the opportunity to visit both and to lecture at both universities, perhaps more at Oxford than at Cambridge. They are tremendous assets in the traditions of excellence they bring to institutions worldwide. During the time I was chancellor of Duke University, I tried to start a formal exchange program with the English universities; it turned out that this was not possible at the undergraduate level because the British students are required to spend a certain number of nights sleeping within a prescribed radius of their university, and thus cannot be physically away over a period as long as a semester. Another consideration was the considerable expense for the student. I have visited friends in England on numerous occasions, especially the internist Dr. John Lister, author of the monthly column "By the London Post" in the *New England Journal of Medicine*, who lives in Beaconsfield, near Heathrow.

In 1992 Dr. Khairy Samra, dean of the Cairo medical school, invited me again to Egypt as his guest and as the guest of President Mubarak. I could bring a delegation of about twenty-two other people to go with me. All we had to do was to travel to Cairo at our own expense, and then we would be the guests of the Egyptian government for two weeks thereafter. The principal reason for the trip was that the Egyptian government wanted to thank me for my efforts to bring the linkage with the national Library of Medicine to Cairo. As of today, I don't know how much of the library system has materialized. However, the trip was very successful in other ways. Some of us rendezvoused in London before taking the British Airways flight to Cairo. In London, the Hotel Lanesborough on Hyde Park (a former hospital), which is managed by Caroline Hunt of the Texas oil clan, had just opened; Caroline was in our delegation, along with her friend Charles Simmons. Since there were several members of our delegation flying with us, I did not know whether to book first class, business, or tourist class for the leg between London and Cairo; I tried to guess which members of the delegation would pay their way in which class. I decided to book myself in business class to be in the middle. Somewhat to my surprise, Caroline Hunt and her escort turned up in the last row of tourist class. The delegation was a distinguished and varied group and included Mr. Frank Barker, a Duke alumnus and corporate vice president of Johnson & Johnson, with his wife; Dr. Ruth Bulger and her husband, Roger Bulger, president of the Association of Academic Health Centers; Mr. John Colloton, CEO of the University of Iowa Hospitals, and Mrs. Colloton; Mrs. Esther Coopersmith, a noted Washington leader; Mrs. Caroline Rose Hunt, an international business woman; Mrs. Rebecca Matlock, Duke alumna and wife of U.S. ambassador to Moscow; Dr. James E. Mulvihill, president of the Juvenile Diabetes Foundation, and Mrs. Mulvihill; Richard W. Riley, a Duke Endowment Trustee and former governor of South Carolina, and Mrs. Riley; Mr. Norb Schaefer Jr., a Duke University trustee and Indianapolis businessman, and Mrs. Schaefer; Dr. and Mrs. Dale Shaw, both

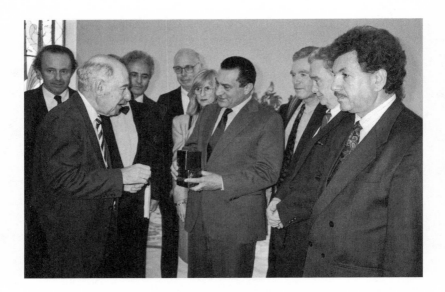

30   Visiting Egypt in 1992 as guests of President Mubarak and Dean Khairy Samra
of Cairo University. (L–R): Dr. W. G. Anlyan; President Mubarak; Dr. Ralph Snyderman, chancellor of Duke Medical Center; Mr. John Colloton, CEO of University
of Iowa Hospitals; aide to President Mubarak. From personal archive of author.

leaders of alumni of the Duke medical and law schools; Mr. Charles Simmons, a retired oil executive; Dr. Ralph Snyderman, chancellor for health
affairs at Duke, and Mrs. Snyderman; and Mr. Louis C. Stephen Jr., vice
chairman of The Duke Endowment, and Mrs. Stephens.

Dr. Samra and his staff met us at the airport at midnight on a Sunday to
get us through passport control and all the other official business, and we
were then loaded onto a bus that took us, with police escort, across Cairo to
the Mena House, where I had suggested we be lodged. The airport in Cairo
is on the east side of the city, and therefore we had to go—around 12:30
or 1 A.M.—all the way across town to the west side, where the pyramids
are located. The Mena House is located at the foot of the pyramids (this
is where Churchill and Roosevelt met with Stalin at the Cairo Conference
in 1942).

The next day, we were granted a very special two-hour audience with
President Mubarak at his official residence. The president was charming
and very cordial. On the second night in Cairo, Dr. Samra had most of
the Egyptian cabinet and the national legislature present at the Sheraton

Hotel at a massive, elegant reception for all of us. He also had arranged for the presence of the best belly dancer in Cairo, who had obviously been tipped off about my Egyptian connections, because she picked me out of the crowd to dance on the floor with her, as everybody cheered us on.

Then we were taken to Aswan, from where we went on to Abu Simbel; on our return, the governor of Aswan had a huge dinner party for us. Included in the tour was a visit to Alexandria, where I took the whole group to see my old school, Victoria College. Then the governor of Alexandria had a formal luncheon for the entire group. We ended up on the Red Sea at Sharm el Sheikh. We were supposed to board a boat to cross the Red Sea to another resort, but the water was very rough and the original boat that had been assigned to us had a fire in the kitchen. Therefore, we were put on a smaller boat. Thirty minutes out, it became apparent that the boat was not up to the rough water, so we returned to Sharm el Sheikh. Then we were off to Cairo for our trip home.

The travels that I undertook as head of the Duke Medical Center over the years were all personally enriching and gratifying. They were also indicative of the growing reputation of Duke University and its Medical Center, which were accorded great respect in the countries we traveled to. Even when there were difficulties and frustrations, there was a real exchange of ideas and impressions, and much good work was accomplished.

14

TRANSITIONS: ON PRESIDENTS
AND CHANCELLORS

W HEN I GOT to Duke in 1949, the new Duke president was
A. Hollis Edens. As a young resident, I knew very little of
what went on at the university; what's more, I did not have
the time during eighteen hours a day spent in surgery to worry about it.
The only time I got into university affairs was in the early fifties, when Wilburt Davison was trying to persuade the university to award Vice President
Richard Nixon an honorary degree. Davison had asked over the hospital
loudspeaker system that everybody on the Medical School faculty go to
the faculty meeting and vote for Nixon. Many of us had not had time to
change for the meeting, so we went with our white coats covering the green
operating room outfits. This, of course, clearly marked the faculty of the
Medical School as being the pro-Nixon group. It was a very turbulent university faculty meeting, and the decision was put off for a few weeks, when
a second faculty meeting was called to take up the matter again. At that
time, however, the request was made over the hospital loudspeaker system
that we all go to the faculty meeting but to be sure not to wear our white
coats. That became a joke on the campus. After that, whenever I went to
the university campus I always made sure that I did not wear my white coat.
So as a young man I had very little contact with the university administration, except as people needed surgical care, when I was called on to render
my services.

When President Edens resigned in 1960, Deryl Hart, who was my boss
as chairman of surgery, was offered the acting presidency of the university

because he was so highly regarded by the university faculty as a fair-minded statesman.

In 1963 a search committee was appointed to find a permanent president of Duke University to succeed Dr. Hart, and they recruited Dr. Douglas Knight from Lawrence College, Wisconsin. (In the meantime, Dr. Hart had gained such respect from the faculty and trustees of Duke University that he had been made full president, with all the honors due.) I had occasion to meet Doug Knight before he signed on the dotted line, and we got along very well. In the six years of his presidency, we became the closest of friends and neighbors. President Knight was kind enough to let me purchase three acres of land just to the west of the area designated for the Duke president's house on Pinecrest Road, a new area of development on the west side of N.C. route 751. Here I built my final home in Durham. Also in the course of our friendship, I persuaded Doug Knight, along with Bud Busse, to buy property on Kerr Lake for second homes that we could use on weekends and vacations.

Doug Knight was and is a humanist, but he was too gentle a person to deal with the turbulent sixties and the Vietnam turmoil on campuses across the country, including Duke's. Doug always wanted to go to bed at night thinking that he had pleased 100 percent of the people he had dealt with during the day. Unfortunately, this was not possible in that era (or in any other). It also was not much help to have as chairman of the Board of Trustees Wright Tisdale, then legal counsel for the Ford Motor Company, who was not a very supportive individual. Every time he had his problems with Henry Ford or the second-in-command who was running the company, he would call and take it out on Doug Knight. In many ways I was the supporting physician to Doug Knight, and on some occasions I arranged for him to be admitted to the hospital just to get some rest from the day-to-day problems of running the university.

Perhaps Doug's downfall started when he gave the go-ahead to a contract for building the president's house on Pinecrest Road. He had been unhappy with the traditional house provided for Duke presidents on the West Campus near the traffic circle, because of the proximity to the student disruptions and all the noise that went with them. He approved construction of the new house without clearing the budget and all the particulars with the executive committee of the trustees. When they found out that it would cost around three-quarters of a million dollars, it provided fuel for those who had been lining up to try to dismiss Knight as ineffectual. I can remember occasions when I was with some of The Duke Endowment trustees when some of them, especially Thomas Perkins and Marshall Pickens, would take Barnes Woodhall and me aside to try to persuade us to help them get rid of Doug Knight. Neither Woodhall nor I would bite on that issue, and we were both supportive of Knight to the very end.

In the meantime, Barnes Woodhall had become the first chancellor of Duke University. This came about when, at a meeting of the executive committee, Doug Knight came in with his appointment book and showed the committee all the appointments that he had and all the matters that he had to take on. He persuaded the committee that he was really doing a two-person job and that he needed a chancellor, a title that had been vacant since Duke President Flowers had relinquished it in the late thirties. By unanimous consent, Barnes Woodhall was appointed to the post, and I earnestly believe that in those days he was very helpful to President Knight. But it was too late; the damage had been done. Doug Knight finally resigned and took a job with RCA, leaving the president's office in the Allen Building empty for almost a year while a search committee sought a successor.

During this interregnum Barnes Woodhall, in his wisdom, worked very closely with Charles Huestis, who had become the vice president for business and finance, and with Marcus Hobbs, who was then the provost. They called themselves the "troika," and as such made and expedited many decisions.

I was appointed to the search committee for the new president, and it was my pleasure to be in the group that finally selected Terry Sanford, although I have a suspicion that he had the support right from the start of trustees such as Charles Wade of Winston-Salem and Mary Semans, who had known him for many years, particularly when Terry was governor of North Carolina. Some of the runners-up on the short list included Bud Busse and Bill Bevan. Bevan at that time was provost of Johns Hopkins University, a position similar to one he had held at the University of Kansas before that. Busse was chairman of psychiatry at Duke.

Terry Sanford arrived with a completely different philosophy from Doug Knight's. A born politician, Sanford did not feel he had to please more than 50.1 percent of the people he saw on any given day. It did not seem to bother him when people disagreed with him. He was a remarkable person, and I really enjoyed working with him over a period of sixteen years. He was a rather unorthodox university president in that he did not follow the usual academic logic of going from A to Z and coming out with the decision that you would expect.

And it never bothered him if he lost. One classic example of that was his support for the project of bringing the Nixon Library to the Duke campus. I was spending a few days' vacation at my house in Beech Mountain, in western North Carolina, when the phone rang about 9 A.M., and there was Terry Sanford. We went through the usual pleasantries for the first minute, and then he pointed out that he was trying to get the Nixon Library to commit itself to coming to the Duke University campus, and after about five minutes of telling me all about it, he asked me to call two of the Medical School members of the executive committee of the Academic Council before a meeting at 9:30 A.M. to persuade them that this was a good move. I indicated to Terry that not only would it be difficult to locate these people in the ten minutes before the 9:30 meeting, but even more to persuade them of the virtues of having Nixon thus honored by Duke in that short a time, since they were both liberal Democrats. I had not forgotten what had happened to the honorary degree for Nixon in the fifties. Ultimately, the Academic Council turned down the request for the library. My dear friend Alex McMahon, who was chairman of the Board of Trustees, came to Terry's support, but it was too little, too late. The Academic Council censured Alex McMahon for trying to establish the library without first getting the faculty's approval, but Terry Sanford came through unscathed.

It should be noted that in Terry's initial telephone call to me about the Nixon Library I admired the fact that Terry, a traditional Democrat, had put aside party politics and was thinking of Duke University's future.

At one point while he was running for the Democratic Party presidential nomination, Terry suffered chest pain in New Hampshire, and the question was whether he had coronary artery disease. I got our mutual friend, philanthropist Walter Davis, to agree to use his Learjet to go up to Boston to bring Terry Sanford back. I took along Dr. Robert Whalen, the most senior cardiologist in the Private Diagnostic Clinics, a nurse from the cardiac care unit, and resuscitation equipment. What I had not banked on was that Walter Davis would accompany us on the plane; his large girth occupied two of the seats at the rear of the plan. At Logan Airport, Terry insisted on walking out to the plane rather than using a wheelchair, since he was being monitored by the press. He puffed out his chest and walked in as erect a posture as possible. I took all the precautions I could think of.

I contacted the cardiologists at Yale, Philadelphia, and Richmond in the event we had any difficulty en route and had to make emergency landings at their respective airports. Nothing untoward happened. Bob Whalen took Terry to Duke Hospital immediately and gave him a clear bill. It had been a false alarm. At that time, I did not know that Terry had a bicuspid aortic valve, which years later developed subacute bacterial endocarditis and had to be replaced. Unfortunately that episode occurred following a dental extraction at a time he was nearing the end of his senatorial election campaign and gearing up for his reelection campaign. Terry lost the race. He was never one to let one loss interfere with all of the other interests he had on the national, regional, or state scene. He was always bubbling with new ideas.

Terry Sanford and I had a wonderful relationship. As a matter of fact, Ken Pye (and subsequently Jack Blackburn, who succeeded Pye as chancellor), Provost Fred Cleaveland (and later Bill Bevan), Charles (Chuck) Huestis, and I used to meet weekly—we called ourselves the "forceps," in contrast to the "troika"—to make university-wide decisions, while Terry took care of the world outside. Also sitting in the meetings was Eugene McDonald, general counsel of the university, since we gradually became a much more legalistic institution, along with every other university, but we didn't change the name of the "forceps." If we disagreed within our little group, we took the matter to Terry Sanford for resolution, and sometimes matters were resolved in my favor, sometimes not. But no one was anyone else's boss, except for the president of the university.

One occasion I remember when we had a little difference of opinion was when the street behind the Medical Center bordering on Sarah Duke Gardens, collapsed. Chuck Huestis wanted me to foot the entire bill of $1.2 million for rebuilding the street, but the reason it had collapsed was because they had created a second lake in the gardens to prevent the flooding of the older pond, which caused the goldfish to spill all over the lawn. I had nothing to do with the go-ahead for that second pond, so I did not see why I should pay for the collapsed street. It was rumored that Isobel Drill, a trustee, had pushed for the second pond, so I was willing to be a good sport and foot half the bill. And that is how the matter was resolved.

I had the privilege of working closely with Terry Sanford not only in the university–Medical Center relationship but also with the external environment, in our relationships with Raleigh and Washington, as well as with other components of the university. Periodically, we went to Washington together to meet with North Carolina's senators and the congressional delegation in regard to matters at the national level.

Terry called me in one day and asked me if I would help him raise the money to air-condition Duke Chapel, and I agreed. The next day I picked up the morning paper to find out that I was chairman of the committee to raise $3 million to air-condition the chapel, which we did rather easily. One-third of the $3 million came as the result of a visit I made to the College of Methodist Bishops at Lake Junaluska, in western North Carolina. I must admit that I felt somewhat out of my league. I had never had a strong relationship with theologians, other than a handful of colleagues at Duke whom I admired. They included deans of the Divinity School since 1949, as well as my good friend, Jim Cleland, dean of the Chapel.

Terry Sanford's biggest contribution to the Medical Center was his support of just about everything we did or planned to do. I never had any problems with the Duke University Board of Trustees, and I feel that this was probably because of three key people: one was Terry Sanford himself. Once he had been briefed on what we wanted to do and felt that it made good sense, he was fully supportive.

In 1982, when Ken Pye decided that he wanted to relinquish the chancellorship of the university, a search committee was appointed to look for a new chancellor. I deliberately stayed away from getting my name on the list because I was very satisfied with running the Medical Center, and we were having a fulfilling (and demanding) time getting Duke into the forefront of academic medicine. Terry Sanford called me in one day and said that there were six people on the short list, two of them from the Medical Center. Before he told me about the two, he asked me if I was willing to become the chancellor. If I was, he would make sure that that came about. He also said that he had talked to Alex McMahon, and they thought that I could have the inside track to become president of the university after Terry's retirement. I thanked Terry profusely and told him that I really did not want to be the number 2 man in operations in any segment of the university or in the total university, that I liked being the number 1 person in the Medical Center. I did not tell him that I did not much cherish the idea of working with non–Medical Center academic faculty because I was used to the action-oriented faculty in the Medical Center, who worked long hours and seldom took sabbaticals or long vacations.

Terry then revealed that the two names from the Medical Center on the short list were Dr. Robert Hill, chairman of biochemistry, and Dr. Keith Brodie, chairman of psychiatry, and he asked me for my thoughts about each one. I told him that Bob Hill was a renowned biochemist, a member of the National Academy of Sciences, but that probably Keith Brodie had a broader vision of the university since he had served several terms on the executive committee of the Academic Council and seemed to enjoy university affairs and dealing with the university faculty. Terry appointed Keith Brodie chancellor. This whole transition took place two or three years later than it should have because Terry's presidency was extended by three years with the support of Charlie Wade, Mary Semans, Alex McMahon, and members of the trustees' executive committee.

Much to my surprise, in the late fall of 1988 Duke University president Keith Brodie invited me to his office and said that he had discovered that he was so involved in the internal affairs of the university that he needed a teammate who would take care of the institution's external affairs. This was just the opposite of the way Terry Sanford ran things: Terry Sanford took care of the world outside while his chancellor took care of the affairs inside the university. Keith persuaded me that he seriously wanted me to be his chancellor, running the external affairs of the university. I swallowed his bait hook, line, and sinker, until I got his proposed write-up of the job description of the chancellor's role, which was labeled "chancellor for external affairs." I objected to this and said that my understanding when I said I would be willing to move from the Medical Center to the Allen Building was that I would be chancellor. P. J. Baugh, vice chairman of the Board of Trustees and Alex McMahon, former chairman of the board, were doing the negotiating, and Keith Brodie finally agreed to my request. However, he did not tell me that he would not relinquish anything substantive when I moved to the Allen Building.

I had some fine offices right across the hall from the president's office, and was able to move not only Joyce Ruark, my long-time administrative assistant, and two junior secretaries but also Janet Sanfilippo and John Thomas—both of them active in fund-raising—to offices on the first floor of the Allen Building for additional support.

Frankly, my relationship with Keith Brodie was a puzzle to me. When Bud Busse retired from the chair in psychiatry, I had appointed a search committee, chaired by Joe Wadsworth and Dan Tosteson as vice chair. They had over one hundred names to choose from, and they presented me with their top candidate, a man at the NIH who was in his fifties. I was unhappy about recruiting an individual of that age who was not in the mainstream of psychiatry, so I thanked the committee and took the book with the resumes home with me for a weekend. I went though the whole book and identified Keith Brodie as the kind of candidate I like to see at Duke. He was thirty-five years old, which meant that he had his career ahead of him. He was an assistant professor at Stanford and did not have tenure, which meant that he was more readily available, although that was not a problem with me because I thought that we could recruit anybody we wanted. He had also become the secretary of the American Psychiatric Association, which meant that he had some national recognition, and his field of research was biological psychiatry and not the traditional psychotherapeutic type.

I invited Keith, and subsequently Brenda Brodie to come on two or three visits to Duke, and we were able to persuade him to become Bud Busse's successor. The criticism I had from some of the other chairs was that he was too young and that he would be in the palm of my hand and would not stand on his own in terms of taking positions that would be good for psychiatry. This proved to be wrong. He seemed to be a team player as well as a good chairman for his department. He was elected to the Academic Council and subsequently to the council's executive committee. Anytime I had a VIP patient I always went through the chairman of the appropriate department, and all the psychiatric problems of trustees, their families, and VIPs were sent to him.

I was pleased to support him to be Ken Pye's successor as chancellor, and when the search committee to select Terry Sanford's successor was appointed in 1985, I also supported Keith as president. What a nice situation it would have made when one of my "favorite sons," whom I had brought to and reared in the Medical Center, would become president of the university. My pleasure at his appointment was genuine, but over the ensuing years, it had become distant and strained.

So I was much relieved when The Duke Endowment and Mary Semans, the chair of the board, offered me the position of a trustee succeeding Frank Kenan, who had just retired from The Duke Endowment. I became chancellor emeritus of Duke University in 1990, after two years of doing my best to make it a decent job as chancellor. My staff and I moved our offices to the tenth floor of the First Union Building at Erwin Square, a new office building not far from the Medical Center. There we worked for five years, next to Gene McDonald and the Duke Management of Assets Company. Subsequently, our offices have been in the Medical Center Library, courtesy of Chancellor Ralph Snyderman and Vice Chancellor Bill Donelan. The Endowment marked a new era in my life, and I have enjoyed directing my energies into its wide-reaching and important work.

15

EFFECTING CHANGE BEYOND DUKE

WHEN I WAS first elected a trustee of The Duke Endowment, I remember looking at the areas of support in health care and child care—or hospital care and child care, as they were then called. It was "hospital care" because, according to the 1924 will of James Buchanan Duke, hospitals were the emerging central focus of health care in the two states to which the endowment's activities are confined, North and South Carolina. The hospital was just changing from a place to go and die to a locus for cure or improvement of patients with major illnesses. "Child care" meant mainly the support of orphanages in both states; at the time, orphanages were still filled with parentless children awaiting possible adoption.

With regard to hospitals, the prevailing attitude of the endowment's trustees for many years had been, "Who knows better than the hospitals themselves what they need? Let them apply for what they need, and if it's legitimate and comes from a nonprofit organization, we will do the best we can to help with as much money as we can." There was no specific program put forth by the trustees as areas for support. With regard to child care, each orphanage was routinely awarded a grant, even though we had come to an era in 1991–92 when there were very few real orphans; the children in orphanages today are abused, unwanted children, many with one or both parents at home. As children's needs changed, we needed to reevaluate our support of institutions that claimed to serve them. In my view, both of the endowment's approaches needed to be changed.

Obviously, I had to move rather slowly because the grand old father of the policies on hospital and child care was Marshall Pickens, for whom I had the utmost respect. He, along with Tom Perkins, had been on the executive committee of the Duke University Board of Trustees that saved my skin when Doris Duke and Dr. Davison were trying to fire me. But over and beyond that single episode, I had a real fondness for Marshall and we had been friends for many years. As Marshall faded out of the trusteeship just before his death, some of the older guard of the staff who had been supporters of the traditional approach to the hospital awards were also retiring. With Eugene Cochrane coming in as the director of the hospital care section, now under the chairmanship of Russell Robinson, we were able to change hospital care to "health care" and to broaden the number of beneficiaries to include other health components. We have come from just 165 hospitals in the Carolinas to many much broader programs and a larger group of potential beneficiaries.

I think I was also instrumental in changing the direction from "bricks and mortar," that is, grants for construction projects, to programmatic support. The exception was small rural hospitals, where we could be convinced that they had exhausted every other source for bricks and mortar before coming to The Duke Endowment. There is no sense, in an era of development offices created to raise money and tax-exempt bonds, to using rare private dollars from the endowment for construction grants. So we announced to the hospital community of the Carolinas that we were moving toward programmatic support. We also gradually began supporting programs in preventive care and children's health, as well as primary care, constantly looking at areas that we should be considering.

We will, for example, look at children with vision, hearing, dental hygiene, and potential skin problems (issues that can be well approached through the school systems). Durham Health Partners were willing to establish an initial study, which has served as our "laboratory" for such programs. In the first few months of looking at problems of vision, with a grant of $100,000 from the Lions Club, we discovered that 1,225 out of approximately 14,000 children in Durham have moderate to serious vision problems that have gone unchecked. Obviously, improvement in vision will have a positive impact on the education of these children.

For a number of years, when I was head of the Medical Center, I tried to get the trustees of The Duke Endowment's hospital and child care sections interested in what I called "physiologic orphans," children whose parents or single parent may still be alive but who are essentially so isolated from those parents that they are, functionally, orphans. I never got anywhere with this initiative, but I notice that the term "physiologic orphans" is creeping into discussion more and more; and there is more attention currently to preventive programs including child abuse. While there are still orphanages, and they are still filled with unwanted, abused children, we should do something when these kids are a lot younger to identify the potential for later problems. I am equally concerned about the fact that there is a large group of children over the age of thirteen who are high school drop-outs, a quarter of whom are allegedly involved in criminal activity within four years. My questions are: When did they go bad? Were they already in difficulty before they dropped out of school? Is the cause genetic? I doubt that criminality among the young has a genetic cause, so the questions then turn to the child's environment, especially the lack of strong family life: when did the problems start in childhood, and what could have been done to get them corrected? One of the things we lack in our society today is the strong family component that prevailed in the past. Parents today are far too permissive.

Under the current leadership of The Duke Endowment, our old hospital and child care sections have changed substantially in the past decade, with a view to looking at the future rather than maintaining a status quo. Under the current leadership of Rhett Mabry in child care, these changes are being made very effectively. Mabry is the son of a Duke medical alumnus, Ed Mabry, an obstetrician-gynecologist in Greensboro, and Rhett himself is a graduate of the Health Administration Program at Duke.

In 1992 Governor Jim Martin had asked me to head up a program to develop a "Healthy Carolinians" concept for the state of North Carolina. Over two years, with the help of Thad Wester, as my vice chairman, and about thirty-five other volunteers, we developed a document for preventive health care for the state. The program was to be supported by the N.C. Department of Health and Human Resources in the state budget; Governor Jim Hunt reappointed me on two more occasions to chair the task force, and I worked on the project till about 1998, when I asked to be relieved. In the meantime, the state government did not come forth with any money. The Duke Endowment and the Kate B. Reynolds Foundation, which supported the original study, funded the project from the initial concept to its development. When the state did not support the program at the local level, The Duke Endowment, believing this an important concept that should be put into effect, stepped in; it has supported sixty such programs across the state of North Carolina, including the one in Durham.

Other areas I am interested in promoting include collaboration among two or more of the academic medical centers, rather than continuing the traditional adversarial relationships. A few years ago I had suggested that Duke and the University of North Carolina consider building a single children's hospital, because I could not foresee the need for two children's hospitals eight miles apart. Unfortunately, for a variety of reasons, this did not come about. Duke has a new children's hospital health care wing; the University of North Carolina, wanting to renovate beds that would also be available for adult occupancy if needed, did not want to participate. But the way of the future will be much greater collaboration and cooperation among the teaching hospitals.

The use of telecommunications is another area in which I have been very interested, particularly to help physicians and nurse practitioners living in isolated rural areas gain access to information and help, especially after the usual business hours, on weekends and nights. The Carolinas Medical Center in Charlotte, which already has an extensive network in North and South Carolina, would be ideal to test such programs. Another test site could be the Duke University Health System, with its large network of hospitals and clinics. But these projects have not yet been defined, and the technology still needs improvement and lower costs.

Currently, Duke has some telecommunication linkages with Saudi Arabia, but there the recipients are able to pay for it. We need to see if we can get these linkages adapted to the situations in rural North and South Carolina. The linkages could be for education, continuing education, and on-line assessment of clinical studies. For example, an EKG can be transmitted very easily so that a cardiologist at a medical center can look at it at the same time as the physician in the rural area. With the adaptation of X-rays to digital processing, X-ray scans can now be transmitted in a similar way. I am sure there is the technology to transmit microscopic biopsy slide collections, as well. These are all exciting possibilities that need to be examined for the future.

I am also interested in the use of computer chips, with the entire medical history of individuals carried in a dog tag or some similar vehicle on everyone's body, wrist bracelet, or a card similar to a credit card. This would be particularly useful for the children of migrant families. As it is, when these children get sick, the health care facility they go to has to start the patient history from scratch for each visit. It would even be useful for me when I am seen in a variety of our clinics as a patient. I would not have to recite my past history and the list of all my current medications.

While The Duke Endowment is an excellent vehicle for supporting and, in some cases, helping to shape the provision of health care in the Carolinas, a number of other groups are also keeping me occupied with questions of health care and biomedical research. One of them is Durham's City of Medicine program.

When my family and I first moved to Durham, it was basically a mill town, home of American Tobacco, Liggett & Myers, and Erwin Mills. But as these businesses shrank, moved away, or closed entirely, Durham needed to find another focus for its energies—and its image. Given the increasing importance of its hospitals and research programs (Duke University Medical Center is the largest single employer in town), Durham decided to dub itself "City of Medicine." Spearheading the effort was the City of Medicine program, begun in 1981 and long headed by the prominent Durham surgeon James E. Davis. I was a founding member of the program, and in 1998, after the death of Dr. Davis, I was asked to succeed him as chairman.

Over the years the City of Medicine program has concentrated on two different efforts. One consists of naming outstanding citizens as "ambassadors" of the City of Medicine: thus the eminent historian John Hope Franklin and the popular health-field writers Joe and Teresa Graedon are ambassadors who carry the good name of Durham wherever they go. The second effort is the development of awards for outstanding scientists from across the world. This idea originated from Mr. Clea Baker, formerly head of government relations for Burroughs-Wellcome.

The City of Medicine awards were begun in 1988. At the time I thought the $5,000 prize was rather insignificant compared to the Nobel Prize, which awards around $1 million to outstanding medical scientists. It turned out that I was wrong. Nominations for the City of Medicine prize have come from all over the country and a few from abroad. The selection committee, which I chaired until recently, is a national committee, and the awards have gone to some people who later went on to win the Nobel Prize. At first we accepted nominations of people who already had won a Nobel, but we decided to concentrate on people who are likely candidates for that prize. In addition to three awards a year for biomedical science, we have given one or two a year for humanitarian service to the state or the nation. In 1999 we gave two: one to Robert A. Ingram, president and CEO of Glaxo Wellcome, and one to Dr. Charles Watts, the African American surgeon, now retired, who served Durham for over half a century, taking care of those who sought care initially at Lincoln Hospital and more recently at the Lincoln Health Clinic. In 2000 we honored Dr. William A. Cleland, a giant who provided pediatric care for generations of African American children in the Durham community. John Edward Porter, former congress-man from the state of Illinois was honored in 2001. He has been recog-nized nationally for his work in balancing the federal budget, protecting the environment, promoting human rights and securing unprecedented funding increases for biomedical research through the National Institutes of Health.

In the years before Jim Davis died, I had kept trying to persuade the board of the City of Medicine to broaden its interests to take on such projects as Healthy Carolinians for Durham County to coordinate many of the health agencies in the community. In establishing the statewide Healthy Carolinians program, we had hoped that each county would establish its own counterpart; it seemed logical for the City of Medicine board to take up the project in Durham. However, Jim Davis and the board decided they did not have the staff to take it on. At that point, I encouraged Carolyn London, a long-time and very effective community volunteer, to spearhead the effort, and she and her duly created board have done an outstanding job of pulling together all the health agencies working in the community in the Durham Healthy Carolinians program.

Then came a third element: in 1998, when the Duke University Health System bought Durham Regional Hospital, it became apparent that the Foundation for Better Health, Durham Regional's development arm, no longer had a raison d'être because the hospital was now owned by Duke, which does its own fund-raising. Jim Russell, the executive director of the foundation, approached me to see if there might be room to merge with the City of Medicine program.

The Durham Healthy Carolinians/City of Medicine merger was begin-ning to pick up steam, with no obstacles en route, when the Foundation for Better Health issue came up. The Foundation for Better Health had a fairly autonomous board of its own, and it took approximately fifteen months for the constituency of the foundation to convince themselves that they should join in a threesome, and under the name Durham Health Part-ners an expanded organization to oversee the provision of health care for Durham County was born.

We attracted a two-year planning grant from The Duke Endowment, at the level of $98,000 a year, to see what health programs should be incorpo-rated into Durham Health Partners. That planning grant started in March 1999, and we have taken on some interesting challenges in addition to get-ting organized. The first major project was vision screenings in the Durham schools. We hope to bring in additional programs to look at the children's dental situation as well as children's hearing—like impaired vision, defective hearing can be a detriment to children's quality of life as well as to their education. The fourth program I would like to consider is melanoma prevention and skin care, particularly protection from the ultraviolet rays of the sun, which is surprisingly neglected in this country.

The whole issue of the care of the underinsured and noninsured population of Durham County is now coming into focus with Durham Health Partners. My impression currently is that nobody in Durham County goes without health care if he or she manages to get in a door to the delivery system. This is in contrast to Palm Beach County, Florida, where the rich either use local providers or fly out of the airport if they have a serious problem, but where the poor have nowhere to go, particularly if they are not covered by Medicaid. We are very anxious that, when a blueprint for the provision of health care for the underinsured of Durham County is developed, it will be looked at by various community groups; in fact, it should be a very open situation, with meetings in different locales geared to patient input, so that all the aspects of the effort can be assessed. The final solution should be one that the community wants, rather than one that Durham Health Partners wants to impose on the population.

Cardiologist and former Duke Hospital CEO Andy Wallace, during a sabbatical year from his duties at Dartmouth, wrote a very fine paper about the problem of the needy and those who are not covered by insurance. I am using his paper as background not only for the initiatives of Durham Health Partners but also to have The Duke Endowment health care committee see what the endowment should be doing in the Carolinas to promote a better look at the problem.

Working with Durham Health Partners is somewhat different from working with the City of Medicine project. I had not realized that the City of Medicine board was regarded as an elitist, academic group. In absorbing both the Durham Healthy Carolinians and the Foundation for Better Health, I became aware of the sensitivities in the community, particularly the African American community, about appropriate representation on both the staff and the board. After my fifty-five years in Durham and at Duke I realized the importance of making sure that we have a diverse, community-wide representation in our programs and in our efforts.

16

FAMILY BONDS

I HAVE LEFT a major part of my story, my family life, till last, though it has been a constant presence, joy, and occasional distress, through all my activities as a physician and administrator, as a member of the medical community in Durham, the State of North Carolina, and beyond.

I was still a medical student at Yale University when I married Catherine Constance Lucier, in June 1948 in New Haven, Connecticut. Connie was born and raised in Nashua, New Hampshire. Her father, Alvin, was a prominent lawyer in Nashua and a staunch Dartmouth alumnus. Catherine Lucier was Connie's mother; she was a very formal person, and until her last decade in a nursing home in Greensboro, I didn't dare call her anything but Mrs. Lucier. In due time she became less stiff in our relationship and I could call her by her first name; she died of a malignant brain tumor. Unfortunately she had suffered from bouts of depression, an illness that all four of her children inherited, in their case to a more serious degree. The Luciers were devout Catholics, while I had no strong inclination toward religion of any kind. At the time of our courtship and marriage I did not appreciate the continuing negative impact this difference would have on our relationship.

Mr. Lucier was a heavy cigarette smoker. In January 1953, while I was in Williamsburg at the Markle selection meeting, Connie had been visiting her parents in Nashua. I got an emergency call asking me to go up there as soon as possible because Mr. Lucier was very ill and getting rapidly worse in the Nashua hospital. His physicians were puzzled about the etiology of his illness. He was fifty-three years old.

I flew from Richmond to Boston and drove to Nashua. At the hospital, he appeared to be deeply jaundiced and semicomatose. Could it be hepatitis? It was immediately apparent that he needed to be transferred to one of the teaching hospitals in Boston. The next day, I took Mr. Lucier by ambulance to the Peter Bent Brigham Hospital, where he died within twenty-four hours. I persuaded the family to grant permission for an autopsy. I cranked up my courage and watched the postmortem examination. Over my five years of marriage I had gotten to like Mr. Lucier and thought he was a very decent and caring human being, if somewhat henpecked.

Much to everyone's surprise, the cause of the jaundice became apparent since the liver was riddled with metastatic tumor. Where was the primary? Examination of the lungs revealed the source, a bronchogenic carcinoma that was no larger than a lentil. It had seeded the liver and the brain.

Ironically, it was the same disease that took Connie, in 1998, after a long illness with both emphysema and lung cancer that had metastasized to her liver. During her final year, she had received chemotherapy with some minimal benefit. She too had been a heavy cigarette smoker (along with her sisters). There were times during some of her depressive states that she smoked or puffed on two to five packs a day. She had given up smoking a few years earlier after suffering from emphysema.

Connie was the new secretary of my mentor, Dr. William German, in the Division of Neurosurgery when I met her in 1948. She was then a beautiful young woman: as an undergraduate she had been photographed and appeared on the cover of *Life* magazine. She had been in New Haven visiting her older sister Louise, who was married to Dr. Julian T. Brantley, a resident in ob-gyn at the New Haven Hospital; Louise persuaded Connie to stay in New Haven and maybe look for a job in the Yale complex.

Connie had served during World War II in the Waves, along with her cousin Helen Doyle, who lived in the Lucier home. But she hadn't ever trained as a secretary. Dr. German told Connie that typing with two fingers was acceptable; he was mostly interested in having a warm and intelligent person handle telephone calls, particularly from patients and referring physicians. So Connie got the job.

It was my junior year in medical school and I was living, for the third consecutive year, on the old campus, counseling undergraduate freshmen at Yale. My older brother, John, had gotten married a year earlier. Even my younger brother, Fred, was married, at the age of nineteen, while still an

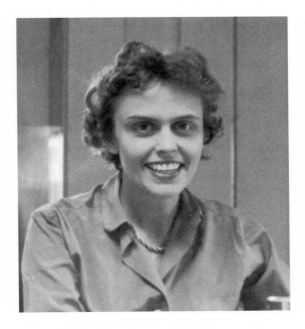

31   Catherine Constance Lucier Anlyan, 1959. Connie was the mother of Bill Jr.,
Peter, and Louise Anlyan. From personal archive of author.

undergraduate at Yale. Here I was twenty-two; was there something wrong
with me? I did not dwell particularly on my disability with arthritis since it
had not impeded my ability to do most activities. In any event, Connie and
I had a whirlwind romance. The convenience of visiting her in the hospital
in my mentor's office and after hours across the street at her sister's home
facilitated the relationship.

A few weeks later I proposed and she accepted, pending my visiting her
family in Nashua. At the time my own parents were living in New Jersey.
They graciously invited us to meet them for dinner one weekend at the
Pierre Hotel in Manhattan. They presented us with two tickets to the hit
Broadway musical *Finian's Rainbow*. My meeting with Mr. and Mrs. Lucier
seemed to go well and shortly thereafter, with a subsidy from my father, a
diamond ring was purchased in New Haven to seal the engagement. Now,
fifty-three years later I wonder why my mother did not offer Connie one
of her many diamonds, which in subsequent years she distributed to her
daughters-in-law.

The marriage was set for June 19, 1948, at a Catholic church in New Haven. In retrospect I realize that I did not take the premarital Catholic instruction very seriously. It was a small wedding; the reception was held at a country restaurant, the Oakdale Tavern, in Wallingford, Connecticut. Those present included the immediate families and our cousins.

Finding a place to live in New Haven in 1948 was a challenge. World War II had ended and the returning veterans coming for varying levels of education at Yale, including residency training at the hospital, was fairly intense. In the preceding weeks like everyone else in the same boat, I scanned the local papers and the obituary columns for potentially available apartments. It was sheer luck that a developer was constructing some reasonably priced garden apartments in East Haven. Along with some resident staff and fellows at Yale–New Haven Hospital, we were able to sign up for one of the two-bedroom apartments. When we left New Haven a year later to go to Durham, my brother John and his wife, Betty, were delighted to take over the apartment, since they were just moving to New Haven.

Our firstborn child was Bill Jr., who arrived on March 13, 1949, at the New Haven Hospital. "Lying-in" and "childbirth without fear" were in vogue, and Connie went through the whole process. Bill was a good-looking baby, robust and happy. The various children's food companies were interested in catering to medical students, so I was able to get a large supply of the ingredients to put in Bill's formula. The carbohydrate was called "Cartose"; it was suggested that 5 percent of the final mixture contain that ingredient. I can recall my thoughts at the time: "If 5 percent is good then perhaps 7 percent is better, especially if we are going to rear a star for the Yale football team." I cringe at the intestinal gas that the extra carbohydrate load produced. I have never quite gotten around to asking Bill Jr. (now over fifty years old) to forgive me.

John Peter (Pete) Anlyan was born a year and a half later on September 26, 1950, at Duke Hospital. He was delivered by Dr. Eleanor Easley, a renowned woman obstetrician who was in private practice in Durham but also had some patients at Duke. "Sis" Easley was a legend in her time; I recall her coming out of the delivery room wearing her OR outfit, complemented by a pair of old army boots, to reassure me that both Connie and Peter were doing well. Pete grew up in the quiet style of a middle child and a Libra (like his father).

Louise Lucier (Weezie) Anlyan was born on August 9, 1953, delivered by Dr. Walter (Buck) Thomas, who in later years became a close colleague

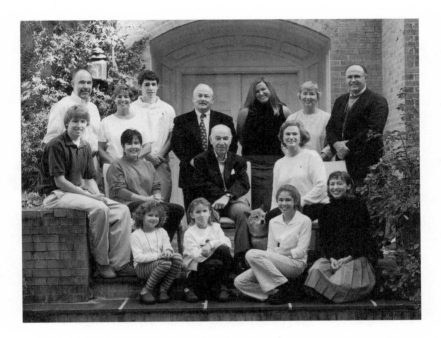

32   The Anlyan children and grandchildren during their visit to Durham on the occasion of Dr. W. G. Anlyan's seventy-fifth birthday, October 14, 2000. From personal archive of author.

and friend. Weezie was the first girl to be born in the Anlyan family for a long time.

Helping to raise my three children has been one of the joys of my life. My only regret as I look back is that I did not spend more prime time with each one of them. The schedule of an intern, resident, and young faculty member in surgery did not provide sufficient family time. Patients and the hospital commanded top priority. Free time for Christmas came by lottery, yet both Connie and the children were forgiving. I am pleased that all three of the children have made prime time with their kids inviolate.

We went through all the usual excitement of raising the children. The children attended Durham Academy (which did not have a high school at that time) and went on to prep school (Westminster in Simsbury, Connecticut, for the boys and Emma Willard in Troy, New York, for Weezie). Graduations and special events were a must, and I attended all of them.

Our happiest vacation times included summers at our cottage at Kerr Lake on the dammed-up Roanoke River on the border of North Carolina and Virginia. We also went as a family to Hawaii in 1964 when I was visiting professor of surgery at Queens Hospital in Honolulu. Other family trips included vacations on the beaches of North Carolina and Rockport, Massachusetts. Occasionally we went to New York City, and I took the family to Broadway musical shows, which they all loved. We would come away with the sheet music of the hit songs of each show. They were played for many years at family gatherings with the children singing around the piano.

Our family friends included the Georgiades, the Busses, and the Parkers. The children of all three families overlapped in ages, and many of them were classmates at Durham Academy. The Busses, and subsequently the Parkers, became neighbors at Kerr Lake. During his presidency at Duke, Doug Knight and his family also had a summer home on Kerr Lake, about two miles away from ours. Our families grew up in a close-knit and long-term group of friends, which provided a stable base throughout their lives.

Bill Jr. received his college education at Duke and Guilford College in Greensboro. Subsequently he graduated from the Duke School of Law. On December 29, 1972, he married Elaine Russos from Raleigh. Bill and Elaine met as volunteers working on Nick Galifianakis's campaign for the United States Senate. They have three children—Sully, Katie, and Matthew. Bill was for a while a development officer at the University of Virginia in Charlottesville and the North Carolina Museum of Art and then served as a vice chancellor at the University of North Carolina in Wilmington. Currently he heads up his own firm in Wilmington, specializing in wealth management.

Pete began his undergraduate studies at the University of North Carolina in Chapel Hill and transferred in his senior year to the School of Drama at New York University. After stints in Hollywood and New York, he moved back to North Carolina to try his acting and production talents here. After running his own children's television show (*Frog Hollow*) at WRAL Raleigh, he moved to the production end of the business. Subsequently he joined the management team of Capital Broadcasting, which assigned him the general managership of the Durham Bulls baseball team. During his five years as manager, he supervised building the new baseball stadium, which has been a key element in the rehabilitation of downtown Durham. Currently he is managing some of the corporation's capital investments in Durham, including the rehabilitation of the American Tobacco Plant across the street from the new Durham Bulls Park. On October 27, 1979, Pete married Harriet (Sissy) Aretakis of Raleigh. Sissy is a first cousin of Elaine Anlyan, and Pete met her at Bill Jr.'s wedding. They have two children — William and Emmy. Pete has also been very active in a series of volunteer jobs in Durham. I am very proud to be known in the Durham community these days as "Peter Anlyan's father."

Weezie went to college at Boston University. She majored in education for disabled children. While in Los Angeles she joined the corporate staff of Century Communications, a cable TV enterprise extending from Australia to the United States and Puerto Rico. In the business, she met her husband, Michael Harris, whom she married on April 22, 1989. Mike became the chief corporate engineer of the company. Eventually they moved to Pound Ridge, New York, next door to their corporate headquarters in New Canaan, Connecticut. They have two daughters, Sarah and Julia. Weezie and Mike were wonderful to have Connie move nearby during her declining years and to help take care of her during her last months, when she was dying from lung cancer.

Connie and I were divorced in 1971, and she moved back to New England to Plymouth, Massachusetts. In 1972 I married Barbara Echols (Bobby), who was in the planning division at the medical center, assisting Jane Elchlepp, the head of planning. I had met Bobby when she was in Washington working for the Association of American Medical Colleges. She had two daughters, Barbra and Laura, who attended Durham Friends School and Durham Academy, and I trust that I was a helpful stepfather to them during those years. Bobby was hard-working and set herself high goals. In her after work hours she studied for an executive M.B.A. from Wake Forest University and subsequently a J.D. from the Law School at North Carolina Central University. Although we separated in 1982, Bobby continued her career and retired as an associate vice chancellor at Duke Medical Center working with Dr. Gordon Hammes, who was in charge of the basic sciences and medical research under my successor Dr. Ralph Snyderman.

In 1985 I met and married Jean Elder Clayton, a Duke alumna, in Miami, Florida. Several months before I had shared a Duke alumni gathering with Terry Sanford in Coconut Grove. The game plan was that it would be a large reception at the Yacht Club. Terry would select fifteen alumni to take to dinner following the reception. I was asked to identify another fifteen to invite to dinner at the Grove Isle Club, where I stayed during my visits to Miami. Before the reception, I had identified only fourteen individuals. In the course of the reception, I met Jean and thought she might be number 15. I did not know that she had checked first with Margaret Rose Sanford to make sure that I was not another "dirty old man" luring her to dinner.

Margaret Rose verified my legitimacy. After dinner, Jean was kind enough to give me her phone number.

In the ensuing months, whenever I was in the Miami area, she joined me. We got into a courtship and on March 30, 1985, we were married on the Howard Hughes Estate in Coconut Grove. (The executive director of the Howard Hughes Institute made an exception to allow this occasion.) Jean was a Duke alumna, class of 1957. She had three children. Skip Virgin, her oldest child, and his wife, Joan, were medical students at Harvard Medical School. (Joan is now a very hardworking pediatrician on the staff of Washington University, Saint Louis, where Skip is a full professor in the departments of medicine and immunology.) John was a champion collegiate tennis player in South Carolina. Karen was the youngest and still trying to find her niche in the world after high school. I have, I believe, been helpful to my all various stepchildren, following their lives and careers with interest and support—Skip and Joan, particularly, with their interest in medicine, where I had some experience and expertise. Jean and I separated in 1994.

In 1997 I married Alexandra (Alex) Hufty. She was born in Washington, D.C., and in her childhood had spent the winter months in Palm Beach. After graduating from the Bishop School in La Jolla, she was in the first class of women at Georgetown University. Among Alex's unique qualifications was breaking the world record in swimming the butterfly stroke as a teenager and becoming an amateur tennis star in her later teens. She played twice at Wimbledon—losing, however, in the early rounds. After fifteen years of married life in Argentina, where she became fluent in Spanish, she returned to the United States, taking on a variety of roles and responsibilities, including working in the Reagan White House. In the early 1990s her mother, Frances Archbold Hufty, assigned her to develop her property Emerald Mountain, adjacent to Beech Mountain. I had known Alex at a distance, as an observer and admirer of her prowess on the tennis courts.

Nick and Ruth Georgiade were kind enough to invite me to dinner with her. It turned out that she also knew something of me, at a distance, for she had been aware of my frequent trips to Palm Beach for fund-raising during the winter season. In December of 1997 we were married in Durham. We have had the good fortune to be able to maintain our home at Duke and Durham during the fall and spring, in Palm Beach during the winter, and Beech Mountain during the summer.

Alex had three children. Her oldest, Alix, a lovely ballerina, died of acute meningococcal meningitis in 1978, before I came into the picture. Miguel

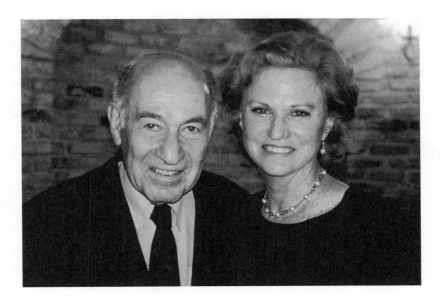

33   Dr. W. G. Anlyan with his wife, Alex, on one of
their recent trips. From personal archive of author.

(Panks), a graduate of Yale and Oxford, is a banker with Deutsche Bank,
living in Munich and Buenos Aires. Sebastian was educated at Dartmouth,
the University of Virginia, and Stanford and is a software computer engineer in San Francisco.

Alex is a stalwart lover of pets and has reintroduced me to the care,
mainly, of dogs. Having lived with a series of beautiful dogs when my children and my stepchildren were growing up, I now find myself quite attached to our dogs. Periodically, I have to remind myself that at one time
my laboratory had the largest number of experimental dogs at Duke Medical Center. I don't think I could return to animal experimentation on such
a scale, given the more personal relationships I have developed with our
current pets.

My "family" life, as I look back on it, has been a full one. Now Alex
and I are engaged mainly with grandchildren. We thoroughly enjoy our
close relationship with my three children and seven grandchildren, as well
as Alex's two sons and her three grandchildren, extending friendship also
to my former wives and my stepchildren. It is somewhat difficult to judge
when to intrude into the prerogatives of our children. When do they really

want the input of grandparents? Still, we find keeping up with birthdays, Christmas, and special events in each one of their lives to be very fulfilling.

Both Alex and I admire families where the parents have been married only once and where marriages have lasted over fifty years—such has been the case with both our own parents. Our current challenge involves staying healthy and productive to enjoy our families for the rest of our lives.

Since December 1997 I have been categorized as "retired" although I am about as busy as I want to be. With telephones, fax machines, electronic mail, and Federal Express, it is much easier to maintain a "global" office year-round, as long as my devoted secretary and assistant, Joyce Ruark, is the anchor at Duke.

Throughout the year, I have numerous daily contacts with my office. Durham Health Partners has required my attendance in Durham one or two days a month, and I have maintained my active interest in the North Carolina Institute of Medicine, which I helped found in 1983. I also commute to my obligations at The Duke Endowment monthly in Charlotte or Durham and attend frequent meetings of Research!America in Washington and elsewhere. Though I relinquished the chair of the board of Research!America four years ago, I remain on the executive committee, the nominating committee, and informally involved in development activities. In Washington, I also serve on the executive committee of the Foundation for Biomedical Research and the executive committee of the Friends of National Library of Medicine. I have remained active in some of the programs of the Association of American Medical Colleges and the Institute of Medicine in Washington.

My top-priority activities, however, are The Duke Endowment—where I am privileged to have just become chair of the health committee, succeeding Russell M. Robinson II, who has now succeeded Mary D. B. T. Semans as chair of the board—and my continuing strong involvement in the growth of Duke University and its Medical Center. My connection with Duke University is somewhat more fuzzy than my work with The Duke Endowment. It involves, on a daily basis, avoiding any interference with my successor, Ralph Snyderman, and his administrative team and yet being available to help whenever asked, particularly with alumni, friends, and patients. My office, namely Joyce Ruark, spends an enormous amount of time in helping new and old patients line up their appointments at Duke. Alex and I do our share and at times host patients from out of town. Frequently patients who are friends stay in our home.

Our lives have been blessed with challenges and achievements, and we relish our continuing activities and our families and friends, who sustain us in more ways than we can say. The one constant in this whole story is change, *metamorphosis*—in ourselves, in the people around us, and in the places we have lived and worked all our lives.

EPILOGUE

LESSONS OF EXPERIENCE

B E H O N E S T W I T H yourself ("To thine own self be true," *Hamlet*). Be your own best critic. If you don't look forward to your job when you wake up in the morning, you may be in the wrong situation.

Be candid—there is no place for half-baked answers or false information. But don't talk too much; instead, be a good listener. It is amazing how therapeutic listening can be for the person who has come to see you. Example: The dean from a neighboring institution called asking for an hour-long meeting the next day to seek my advice on an urgent matter. When he arrived, after the usual brief greeting, he spoke for fifty-nine minutes. As he rose to leave, he thanked me profusely for my advice, which I never got a chance to give.

Keep the clock in your office ahead by a few minutes. I had mine located on the wall facing the visitor. It was not unusual for the individual to apologize for being a little late, adding, "I'll hurry up and tell you why I wanted to see you."

Never sit behind your desk so there is a physical barrier between you and your visitor. Always have a cozy little sitting arrangement in a part of the office where the visitor is on an equal level. I am always appalled when visiting other individuals, especially government bureaucrats, who "hide" behind a huge desk denoting their authority. One of the funniest interviews of my student days was with an assistant dean of the Yale Medical School who was barely five feet tall. He sat on a high chair, and I was on a couch six inches off the floor across from his desk.

Have the courtesy of greeting your visitor outside your door. At the conclusion of the meeting, if time permits, escort your visitor to the door of the office suite.

Do not have the fanciest office in the organization. I always tried to have an office that was smaller and slightly shabbier than the persons reporting directly to me. On one occasion, at a meeting of all the department chairs, they passed a resolution asking me to refurbish my office because they were embarrassed to bring distinguished visitors to see me.

Never be the top wage earner. Do not drive a fancy car—your parking place is well known, and there is no need to show the thousands of other employees and faculty who earn less than you do where you rank economically.

Have an escape door to your office for the rare occasions when you have an unwanted visitor. I recall my administrative assistant coming through the back door to escort me to safety when a former exotic dancer, whom I had never met, showed up in my secretary's office asking to see "the head man." Early in her encounter with my secretary, a revolver fell out of her purse; she was unhappy with the result of some cosmetic surgery, which was actually done at another institution.

Maintain professional proficiency in your basic field, because (a) it keeps you sharply honed to the current state of your discipline by teaching, reading, and going to the conferences in the field (you will not be administering medicine of a bygone era); (b) if you are fired or choose to step down, you have a gracious way out to go back to your intellectual pursuits; (c) it lets you spend time "in the trenches," where you can associate with students, faculty, and employees—most of whom would never make a formal appointment to see you in your office—and remain "one of them," taking your turn on the front line. Throughout my twenty-five years as the head of the Medical Center, I continued to teach surgery and to practice, though the latter dwindled with time. Over the years I have been amazed at the number of former and current employees throughout the university—campus police, barbers, orderlies, nurses, alumni, and younger faculty members—who remember, usually kindly, their associations with me.

Answer your correspondence promptly, within twenty-four hours if possible. Even an acknowledgment of receipt is important. Do not be afraid to refer letters to other individuals if the subject is outside your area of competence; however, let the writer know that you are doing so. There is no embarrassment in saying that the matter is being looked into. Also, there is no need to answer each detail of a lengthy letter, point by point. I have found that a one-paragraph letter thanking that person for the advice and input will often be sufficient to let the letter writer feel he or she has been listened to. One letter I shall never forget was a shaky handwritten note by an eighty-five-year-old former patient, enclosing three one-dollar bills, adding that she did wish to express her gratitude but that it was all she could afford.

Answer your telephone calls by the evening of that day. If you are in a remote part of the world, your secretary can respond by letting the individual know that it will be brought to your attention at your next call-in.

One of the most important components of a successful operation is to have a superb staff—your personal secretary and your administrative staff can make or break you. If you are a CEO, you cannot afford to have any member of your team who is not top-flight. They should be amongst the best paid in the institution for their rank. There is no need to break the rules, but the rules can be changed throughout the institution as necessary. Overpayment beyond established scales leads to other key officers in the organization trying to do the same thing, and this leads to chaos.

If you aspire to be a CEO, avoid being chained to a computerized telephone answering system. Answering machines are acceptable after hours, but working through a maze of impersonal nonhuman messages before you reach a real person is a turnoff. Airlines and other complex businesses can get away with it, but not the office of a CEO.

In selecting senior associates, pick "deciders" who in their daily work can make 95 percent or more of decisions within their responsibility and authority. You do not want a team made up of "messengers" who bring over 5 percent of their decisions for you to make.

Don't be afraid to recruit subordinates who are smarter than you. They will augment the quality of your organization. Lesser individuals will perpetuate mediocrity. Not everyone you select will be a success; expect some failures and disappointments; take them in your stride.

Whenever possible, delegate responsibility, but be prepared to back that person. If he or she erred, talk to them privately but avoid any public embarrassment. If the problem is a recurring one, the individual should be replaced and allowed as gracious an exodus as possible.

Your time as a CEO should be devoted to "tomorrow" and not "today." You should spend your energy on making the institution better for the future. You should not clutter your day with nonpolicy issues that can be managed by junior colleagues. As my former colleague Ken Pye (then chancellor of the university) used to say, sort out the "elephant problems from the peanut problems." I have run into senior colleagues throughout the university who have wasted their time and effort on peanut problems without recognizing the bigger issues. Do not micromanage: once you have delegated, don't backtrack and monitor your colleague.

Make sure that your management team includes a financial manager, a comptroller and budget officer, an office manager, and a legal staff. The latter would be managed and coordinated by one general counsel with direct access to the CEO. In the world of today the general counsel needs the support of a variety of special legal counsels both within and outside the institution.

In dealing with your fellow human beings, accept the fact that 85 percent of the average person is good, 15 percent is bad or could be better. Try to work with the 85 percent that is good; on rare occasions the 15 percent bad is up front and difficult to penetrate or circumvent. In developing a "team," try to match the 85 percent good of each member.

Forgive and forget! We are all capable of making mistakes. Why not erase the memory after necessary acknowledgments and corrections have taken place? There is no sense wasting energy storing and retrieving errors. The one sin that is unforgivable is dishonesty; there should be no room for anyone who cheats either financially or by falsifying results. Occasionally, there may be a suggestion of dishonesty, in which case the individual should be confronted, privately but in the presence of a colleague as a witness. Once, a senior member of the faculty appeared to be shading his travel expenses. In my meeting with him, I said, "If you are going to cheat, cheat big and go to Brazil. There is no room in this organization for nickels and dimes." He never fudged thereafter.

Be kind and gracious to everyone—especially to the lowest-rank employees and the poorest patients. They do not have many choices or options. One of my beloved mentors, on the day of his retirement admonished me as follows: "Be nice to everyone—you never know who's going to be your next boss." He was right. I had been his intern in 1949, his resident till 1955, his faculty colleague to 1963, and his dean until his retirement.

Dr. William G. Anlyan is Chancellor Emeritus of Duke University and a
Trustee of The Duke Endowment. In his half-century of service to Duke, he
has been a surgeon and professor of surgery, Dean of the School of Medicine, and Executive Vice President for Health Affairs. Among his many
honors are the Abraham Flexner Award, the highest honor given by the
Association of American Medical Colleges; the Lifetime Achievement Award
for Duke University Medical Alumni, now renamed in his honor; the Yale
Distinguished Alumni Service Award; the Duke University Medal; the City
of Medicine Lifetime Achievement Award; and the North Carolina Award
in Service, the highest honor the State of North Carolina can bestow.
Dr. Anlyan lives in Durham.

Library of Congress Cataloging-in-Publication Data
Anlyan, William G.
Metamorphoses : memoirs of a life in medicine / by William G. Anlyan.
ISBN 0-8223-3378-3 (cloth : alk. paper)
1. Anlyan, William G. 2. Physicians—North Carolina—Biography.
3. Medical colleges—North Carolina—Faculty—History.
[DNLM: 1. Anlyan, William G. 2. Duke University. Medical Center. 3. Faculty,
Medical—North Carolina—Personal Narratives. 4. History of Medicine,
20th Cent.—North Carolina. 5. Schools, Medical—history—North Carolina.
WZ 100 A612m 2004] I. Title.
R154.A59A3 2004   610′.92—dc22   2004004075